Extreme Rapid Weight Loss Hypnosis for Woman

Say goodbye to the risk of Gastric Band Surgery. You'll find: Gastric band Hypnosisis, mini habits, affirmations, meditations. Burn fat safely and easily

D.R. Nigel Ross

Please consult a licensed professional before attempting any techniques outlined in this book.

By reading this document, the reader agrees that under no circumstances is the author responsible for any losses, direct or indirect, which are incurred as a result of the use of the information contained within this document, including, but not limited to, — errors, omissions, or inaccuracies.

Table of Contents

Introduction

Do you know what's worse than having an oversized body? It is the loneliness that accompanies it. No one wants to date me, I don't blame them. Who would want to love a fat blob? I have no curves, nothing special in my body that attracts someone to love.

My family and friends have accepted me the way I am. They love me and this is the only comforting thing in my life. I have been overweight in the past decade. Maybe they have accepted that I cannot lose weight and love my company. Everyone tells me to stay happy and love my body. How can I? There is nothing there to love. I cannot stand in front of my mirror and say "wow, nice abs". Whenever I enter the shower, all I can think of is how ugly I am. Who would love me? With these thoughts, I tend to pass most of my day sad and depressed.

I have learned to accept myself as I am but this does not cater to the fact that I am fat and probably going to have several diseases. Don't get me wrong, I am no pessimist but science backs me up on this fact. Overweight people tend to catch more diseases such as problems with the heart, arthritis, and even have less life expectancy. I cannot deny that if I do not take my diet seriously, I will be stuck in a wormhole and will be sucked to the abyss. I do not want to die with several diseases, nobody does. My body is in such bad shape that it leads to mental pressure as well. The mental pressure of finding love, mental pressure of the glares that I receive when I walk down the road. I feel enormous pressure when I am in a family gathering. Most of my relatives have seen me skinny in the past and meeting them after many years is no joke. I listen to them for hours telling me how skinny I was (like I never knew about it). My folks tell me about hundreds of weight loss programs and remedies that they deem fit for me. I know they must be genuinely worried about me and are only trying to uplift me from this pit of obesity. But what they do not know that I have tried many things but can never complete the program. There are days when I didn't eat anything and felt happy that I am making progress with the weight loss program and there were days when I just sat down, chugged a whole cola, and ate till my belly hurt. There was nothing in-between. I knew I need some consistency and knew that I had to change my life.

I could not persuade you to lose weight or say that losing weight will help you get the love of your life and you will live happily. I know many people with obesity that live a happy life and have someone to love. The beauty standards are different in different parts of the world. The African male prefers their women fat and chubby. Unfortunately, not all men share the same standards. We live in a society where skinny models have shadowed the fashion industry and beauty is all about being skinny. The twenty-first-century fashion industry is filled with skinny models and the zero-size figure is considered the sexiest and appealing. You cannot force anyone to like you whether you are skinny or fat. You cannot change how they think so there is no use thinking about it. All you can do is to be focused on your health and personal fitness and never force them to love you.

I have known many overweight people fall into depression and anxiety. The anxious mind can do tricks on you and you may tend to overeat. This is a vicious cycle that can pull you towards abomination. I decided to change my life and walk into the path unknown. I made changes to my daily life and started to feel good every day. I trained my mind in such a way that I could love myself and try to reduce my body every day. I did not know how powerful our minds can be. My attitude towards my diet, my body, and my life changed after that.

As William James wisely said, "Human beings, by changing the inner attitudes of their minds, can change the outer aspects of their lives."

To be honest, I am still trying to change and still trying to adapt to my new thinking. Yes, I slack sometimes and eat improperly at days but the positivity of my mind does not let me wander back in the same direction as I was before. I want to share my experiences with you and tell you how your mind can help you change your overall habits and tune your body. How it can change you into a better version of yourself. This book is not only about how you can lose weight. This is about how you can change your thinking and start living a better life – a better life that will bring happiness and prosperity. By reading this book, you will be able to explore the mind-body connections, the role of therapies in your weight loss and positivity in your life, and the role of affirmations in your daily life especially how you see yourself. We will try our best to make this journey as easy for you as possible and will ensure that you get the best insight from the experiences of many professionals.

Chapter 1:

How Does the Mind Work?

Once I realized that I needed to change the way I eat and the way I live my life, I started noticing many changes in my overall life. I was so depressed seeing my body in the mirror and I completely changed how I need to see myself and it was clear what I needed to work on. Instead of thinking that I looked ugly, I started to see the parts which needed to be reduced. I started to focus on the light at the end of the tunnel rather than the darkness that I was in. This wasn't easy and I will tell you this, it will be along and tiring process and you will need to work on it with a positive mindset. You will need to learn how your mind works and how you can reshape your thinking to achieve greatness in your life. Our body and mind share a beautiful connection and we need to learn to listen to them. Our body gives signals to the mind and the mind responds to them within nanoseconds.

Mind/Body Connection

Everyone around you wants to be healthy, intelligent, and successful. We all want to reach a certain level where we can cherish our life. We set some goals in our lives and work to achieve them. When your goal is to lose weight, you will imagine yourself eating less and exercising more – but believe me, losing pounds is way more than this. It is a process that requires high mental capability, resilience, and the ability to control your urges. Yes, the urge to control eating and the urge to look fantastic. In our lives, we are blessed with abundant food and this makes us ignore the signals that we get from the body and eat whenever we want. I remember eating my favorite chocolate pie every day because I liked it so much. When we eat food that we love, it gives positive signals to the mind and we feel good. So good that we forget when to stop. Eating pie became a habit of mine and soon one serving turned into two and after a while, I could not imagine my day without eating almost half of that pie. I did not know when to stop or to think about how it will affect my body.

We, humans, can lose sight of the bigger picture as we always get an appreciation for how we are performing in the world. This means that we can easily lose sight of the bigger picture and find comfort in the support we receive. All of us lose sight of the other level that is waiting for us and the blinders block our view and we do not work for reaching the higher goal. You need to know that each step that you conquer will open new doors of success for you. I never surpassed the initial doors and this made me worried about what the future has stored for me. When someone appreciated my work, I tend to get into the comfort zone and stopped working. The main question that you need to realize is that can you recognize this illusion? We all have been living in the illusion and do not see a way to get past them. You need to see these illusions and see past them. In your life, you will stumble upon different people. People who tend to lose sight of the big goal and will also meet people who are always focused on what they want. Almost sixty percent of the people never see outside the hole they are in. Victims make up for twenty percent of the population. Such people blame others for their demise. More than fifteen percent of people fall into the category of survivors. These people will do the work when they are in trouble and will fight to get themselves in a good position. Only five percent are winners. Those who never lose sight of the main goal. I saw myself in the category of people who were in a pit hole of demise. I never set a goal for myself and this is why my mind always played tricks on me. The road to the winners was a tough one and all I had to do was to prepare my mind so that I could imagine how the body will react. And it reacted positively!

In the Twinkling of an Eye

Whether you believe it or not, your present body is affected by your beliefs and thoughts. Your lifestyle is a combination of your beliefs and thoughts and they are the reason behind your current body type and weight. It is not a matter of right and wrong. You haven't acted wrong or made a mistake but have got unwanted results from the lifestyle you adopted. I did not want to get fat, and I certainly know you didn't as well.

Your behavior and lifestyle are shaped by these skewed thoughts and beliefs. You have changed your thought process in such a way that you didn't even look back at what you were and where you were heading. The phenomenon of self-hypnosis diet is the process of aligning your thoughts to achieve the results you want. With this, you will be able to achieve the bodyweight that you want with the help of your thoughts. Let me take you down the memory lane and help you understand how you ended up in this place. Do you have the bulky body type from childhood, or you got these pounds as time passed? Or maybe you just woke up one day and realized that you have gained a lot of weight. Whatever the reason may be, some factors have created your current body. Some factors are depicted below:

- Food Choices
- Emotional and Economic Background
- Family Influence
- Friends Influence
- Cultural background
- Eating habit
- Self-Criticism

Many other factors also play a role in shaping your beliefs and thoughts and they define your current body type. I need you to turn back time and answer these questions to understand how you have been spending your time till now. Humans learn about eating and food in their childhood and taking some time to analyze ten questions will let you know where you made a mistake and how you can alter your mind to tune your body.

- Did you ever learn about eating mindfully? If yes, then when!
- Did you learn that eating healthy can lead to a healthy body?
- Did you learn what falls into healthy food?
- Did you make your food choices based on the price or nutritional value of the food?
- Did you learn about nutrition and a healthy lifestyle from school or advertisement and what were your beliefs about the body, food, and eating in general?
- What type of groceries did you get while growing up?
- What food items were mostly cooked in the house?
- Did you eat at home or ate fast food more often?
- Did you eat junk food or a good home-cooked meal?
- Did your family ate while keeping nutritional value in mind, or just ate blatantly?

This exercise will help you test your sociocultural and socioeconomic roots and you will be able to gauge if they played a role in determining how you eat and how you see your overall diet. Research conducted in the 1990s showcased that people with sociological problems have more weight-related issues as working-class consumptions patterns were found to be irregular. These consumption patterns are referred to as "poverty level foods". Some food items that fall in this category are canned meats, processed meat, and hot dogs. People with different cultural patterns have also been studied. There dietary pattern and food items were put under the microscope to test how they cook food and how they look at their dietary requirements. It was revealed that cooking with lard and having a diet with increased fried food and high-fat substances increases the chance of greater body fat. These influencers for increased body fat are considered normal as many people generally fall in this class.

Now, we will take a look at how the mind and gut connection works in the adolescent years. In the teenage years, the body goes through different transformations. Many people tend to change their eating habits and you also get encouragement or discouragement for your eating habits. I have been eating less during my teenage years and an aunt of mine told me to consume more if I want my body to be attractive. Wider hips and getting tender breasts were my goal during my teenage years and this affected my eating habits and how I see my food. This was also the time when I learned about obesity and didn't want to fall into this abyss. You also need to ponder over those years and this will help you understand how you have developed your current body. You might also recall the time when you learned about the physical activities and how they affect your overall body type. You need to recall whether you were introduced to the physical activities as part of living a healthy lifestyle or you just saw these physical activities as some unnecessary chores. As you were growing up, you must have realized how mindful you have been regarding your diet and physical activities. It is best you to make notes of how you have been spending your early years.

Your mind can do wonderful things. It can be positive and negative and you need to train it to help you see positive in your life. The next section will focus on how you can boost your belief system and how it can help you overturn your negative habits and turn your life around.

Obesity expands the danger of creating hypertension, diabetes, and metabolic condition, which increment the danger of cardiovascular failures and strokes. Metabolic disorder alludes to various conditions, including stomach weight, high triglycerides, high LDL (awful) cholesterol, hypertension, and significant levels of glucose. After secondary school, you most likely moved away from home. Out of nowhere, you were not, at this point hostage to your family's way of life. Did you become increasingly aware of your decisions, or did you start eating with ignorance? If you went into a cozy relationship, what bargains or understandings in regards to food and physical action did you go into too? Most connections create out of comparative interests, for example, food inclinations and eating styles. Eventually, the relationship incorporates eating examples and inclinations that are an aftereffect of the bargain.

Have your connections supported savvy food decisions and good dieting? Maybe you have encountered pregnancy. Did you figure out how to have a solid pregnancy and sustain a sound infant inside you? Or then again did you include pounds onto pounds? In the wake of conceiving an offspring, did your way of life assist you with recapturing your typical weight or hinder it? If you were dynamic in sports or association games, did your profession or family duties take need and expel these wellness exercises from your daily practice? Did you modify diet and exercise as needs are, or did the weight begin to collect? Did a physical issue, mishap, or sickness happen that upset a customary physical action that was strong of solid weight?

The British Medical Journal conducted an examination which shows that individuals who were overweight in their forties are 35 percent bound to build up a memory issue sometime down the road than those individuals who had ideal weight.

Keep in mind, you didn't do anything incorrectly, yet you have encountered the consequences of living and eating that were steady with your considerations and convictions.

Set Some Ideal in Your Mind

It is best to have some ideal in your mind that you look up to. It can be a celebrity, a friend, or even a coworker. Let me share an example. The September 2005 issue of First for Women incorporated a story and photographs of a lady who went from a load of 280 pounds down to 148 pounds. She depicted seeing her five-year-old child stuck to the window, viewing a local family plays a round of soccer. She thought I realize he needs to play more than anything, however, we would do well to remain inside. She settled on the choice at that moment to change. She recorded the progressions she made in eating, and exercise, commenting that "my inspiration mentor (her child) was there day in and day out."

Her craving to join her child turned into an astonishing inspiration impetus. In the shimmering of an eye, you can place the vitality of your craving and convictions without hesitation, and you are moving yourself to do it. Throughout the years, what has been your reaction to individuals and their remarks about your weight, positive or negative? Did you go out and purchase a decent pair of running shoes, or did you eat to facilitate the enthusiastic inconvenience? Maybe you even took in the last response in your adolescence. Did your mom ever give you a plateful of food to comfort you when you were miserable? These are learned reactions, and they can be unlearned and supplanted with new reactions and examples to make your ideal weight. You ask, "To what extent will this take?" We let you know, "In the glimmering of an eye."

For the second you understand that you need it enough to successfully have it, it is finished. You have quite recently altered the course of a ground-breaking vitality inside you that will currently be guided toward figuring out how to accomplish the outcomes that you need: your ideal weight.

Mind Relearning

It is straightforward how you gained or "learned" to gauge more than your ideal weight. Furthermore, it will be anything but difficult to settle on new decisions, to relearn new examples, and to make new and increasingly refreshing inclinations. How would we learn? We learn by displaying someone else, considering books (like this one), utilizing different possessions, and rehearsing the activities that produce the outcomes we look for. The best and enduring learning includes practice and reiteration. How you practice is especially significant. Imagine for a second that you are a musician. You are practicing for a fabulous orchestra execution in New York City.

Your piece has a portion of five bars that are hard for your fingers to play accurately. There are two different ways for you to rehearse. The principal, which is inadequate, is to play that troublesome section rapidly, again and again, and over once more, ceaselessly playing similar errors, yet trusting your fingers will at last play it effectively. The subsequent method to rehearse, which is consistently effective, is to play the section extremely, gradually, carefully "educating" your fingers how to move, making the "muscle memory" for the right developments, until your fingers have taken in the developments and can play the whole fragment accurately and at the best possible rhythm with little, assuming any, cognizant consideration.

The significant point here is that you are focusing on rehearsing effectively. By being aware of what you are rehearsing, and how you are rehearsing it, you are learning the new examples that are supplanting the old examples. You are rehearsing the movement that delivers your ideal body weight. You, as well, can make "muscle memory" by rehearsing careful (eating gradually, biting completely, gulping the last nibble before you take the following chomp) or an increasingly careful, more slow fork-to-mouth development.

You can likewise rehearse a whole eating style that gets molded as a mind-body memory or realizing, which rapidly gets programmed. As it becomes programmed, you don't need to try as your body will do the task itself.

Train Your Mind Starting Today

These new contemplations start to swarm out those old examples that gave you undesirable outcomes. It is a lot of like going on a garments shopping binge. At the point when you add new garments in your storage room, you make room by throwing the old garments or placing them in a sack for another person. Settling on positive decisions dependent on what you need and placing them as a primary concern, alongside doing your self-hypnosis, will help you serenely embrace all the new examples, practices, and decisions that impact your ideal weight. Relinquish all expectations for a superior past, and continue with what you can do at this moment. As you go ahead creation changes every day, you are gathering an ongoing past that supports giving you the ideal weight you have picked.

It's the game of Choices

Everything is a decision. If you deliberately concur with what you read here and what you hear during the trancework, your psyche says, "Yes!" or "I'll do it for you!" That is, your inner mind, your brain-body, will reflect what you pick and consent to acknowledge or accept. Similarly, as you can pick what to accept, you can pick what to realize. Furthermore, with reiteration and consistency, you are making the educated reactions that immediately become programmed or natural. In this way, the decisions you are making, alongside the considerations and activities you accurately practice, give you the outcomes you want.

Absorb it like a hobby

Hobbies give us the fulfillment of learning new things and consuming our psyches with lovely encounters that lead to a result that likewise satisfies us. Approach your weight reduction exertion as though it were another leisure activity. Entertain yourself with magazines, instruments, and books, maybe even classes and intrigue gatherings. Commit an exceptional region of your home to your interest. Similarly, as different hobbies offer you an invigorating reprieve from work exercises, let your weight reduction leisure activity additionally serve to give you a reviving option in contrast to your activity or work. In any event, when you are grinding away, you may discover awesome approaches to consolidate time and regard for this pastime. The Internet, book shops, libraries, and newspaper kiosks are loaded with reading material for you. You don't have a clue where the least difficult, yet most capably motivating thoughts will come to you. Try not to constrain yourself to diets and notices about weight reduction. Give everything access this world presently serves your diversion. You are making this interest. Appreciate it for yourself solely.

Chapter 2:

Weight Loss & Hypnosis

One of the main researchers that claimed the body and soul are conjoined with each other was René Descartes. His studies showcase that both mind and body are aligned with each other. René later stopped researching on this topic as he considered that the matters of the heart are in the Church's domain. However, he wasn't that only one who studied and researched the connection between heart and mind. The studies of many researchers reveal that the mind and body are different entities but share a close bond. One cannot exist without the other.

Both mind and body are in constant communication with each other. One can influence the others in many ways. A person can feel the connection several times each day. The mind tells the body what to do and the actions of the body are felt by the mind. The sensations of the body and the thoughts of the mind are interconnected. I have been wondering the thought of changing my body for many years but it was in recent times that I realized that I cannot achieve anything by just working on my body. I need to make changes to my thought process, how I perceive things, and need to train my mind to help my body lose weight. Self-hypnosis is a method that influences the body and helps you regain your lost confidence and can also help you shed the extra pounds that are weighing down your life.

Before you can learn the actual method of losing weight by training your mind, you need to learn about hypnosis. I will discuss the origin of the term and this will help you understand the real essence behind this term and you will be able to differentiate between the fact and fiction. The mind-body connection is the heart of this term. The communication between the mind and body is a lossless phenomenon that continues all the time. Your first task is to understand this communication and this will help you to achieve your perfect weight. Learning the thought process behind things is imperative for this process. You will not be able to see them but they will always be by your side. You will not be able to feel every thought that crosses your mind. Thanks to the advancement in technology, we can attach the biofeedback sensors to your body and you will be able to feel all the changes in the body when you think positively or negatively.

Don't get confused, I will simplify it for you. Think of someone you hate or someone who makes you angry. You will start to notice a change in the heart function, change in the nervous system, changes in the blood pressure, and will also feel the muscle tension. These things will be triggered by a single thought. This tells you that the thoughts and ideas make changes in the body. These chemically triggered changes in the body are triggered by your emotions or thoughts. Most of the time a person does not know that the actions are triggered by the thoughts.

Many factors affect your response to your thoughts. The past experiences, your personality, your patterns of response, and even your attachment style can moderate your response to a specific thought. Your body will function according to the response pattern. The repetition of these patterns will embed in your body and you will always perform in a certain manner. To be honest, when I learned about this fact, I was afraid because I just sat on the couch most of the time during the past decade and every response of my body was related to food. When I was sad, my body craved for food. When I was happy, I wanted the same. I genuinely didn't know when I was actually hungry or just fulfilling a never-ending craving. But not all was lost and all is not lost for you as well. The good news is that you can unlearn anything by changing your habits. Self-hypnosis is one of the best ways by which you can unlearn things and replace them with more suitable configurations.

As described at the start of the chapter, the mind and body share a beautiful connection. The thoughts can influence the body and in the same way, the body can influence the thoughts. Some sensations in the body can trigger the thoughts. When you have a dry mouth, you will think of drinking the water. These sensations are not easy to understand and can sometimes confuse a person. Let us take an example of a sad person who has recently gone through a breakup. An emotionally hurt person might get confused between the notions of "I want to eat" and "I need to eat". The rapid weight loss hypnosis focuses on how the mind and body are connected and eliminating such confusion from your mind. Until recently, I didn't know that the subconscious mind is an important part of the daily routine and it controls many actions of our body. When you plan to lose weight, you need to train your mind to give signals to the body that can help you achieve your goal at a faster pace.

What Is Hypnosis

Hypnosis is an extremely successful path for you to talk straightforwardly to the brain of your body (the body-brain or brain-body). It gives you an approach to evacuate any obstructions inside the exchange of your psyche body, so mind-body is sharing precisely what you need in a manner that helps you get a sound weight and live a happy life. Before we go any further, we might want you to finish a short mental exercise that will assist you with starting to find out about the force and the straightforwardness of self-hypnosis. The following are ten "valid or bogus" articulations about hypnosis. Peruse the announcements and marvel, surmise, or choose "valid or bogus" as indicated by what you presently accept about hypnosis.

1- Hypnosis is a very complicated process and if you want to learn it, you have to spend many sessions and follow many instructions.
2- You will have to be hypnotized by a person who knows this trade.
3- The person loses touch with his consciousness when he/she is in a hypnotic trance.
4- The subconscious mind will not know the difference between the imaginary and real worlds.
5- The hypnosis will let you do unwanted things and you may also violate your values in this process
6- People go the stage of trance every day.
7- Hypnosis is also known as self-hypnosis.
8- The process of hypnosis can help you heal your body
9- The body has a language and it cannot be understood.
10-   The process of hypnosis can be used to change the physical responses such as breathing and digestion.
11-Medical hypnosis is similar to stage hypnosis
12-   Sometimes you will not know when you are in a trance

13-   Hypnosis is a mental stage and it just a mental phenomenon

14-   Some people in the world cannot be hypnotized

15-   The hypnosis can be used to give messages from the body to the mind and vice versa

16-   You can easily find thousands of research studies on this topic that can help you evaluate the benefits of hypnosis.

Perusing these announcements is a significant advance. It primes your cognizant brain to be watching out for the appropriate responses all through these pages and your involvement in the sound. (On the off chance that you can hardly wait, the appropriate responses are in Appendix An.) It is critical to respond to altogether any inquiries you may have about hypnosis. The purpose behind this is basic. To have the option to "let go" of any falterings and experience hypnosis, you should have a sense of security and agreeable inside yourself when utilizing the methods introduced on the sound bit of The Self-Hypnosis Diet. The more you think about hypnosis, the more agreeable and sure you will feel utilizing it.

Daydreaming and Trance

Regular encounters of daze are normal. At the point when you are gazing out a window, your eyes are open. They are recording light and shape and shading. The poles and cones in your eyes are reacting, and the optic nerve conveys the data to your mind. You are gazing vacantly at nothing in particular. You are actually "seeing," however you are not really "looking" at what you are seeing. This is a case of an ordinary encounter of a daze. You can likewise gaze with your ears. Eardrums are tympanic. They resemble the heads on drums. They move with the adjustments in pneumatic stress (sound waves). At the point when you are gazing with your ears, you are in fact "hearing" because your eardrum is moving, and the little bones in the ear convey the message along the nerve pathways to the cerebrum, yet you are not "tuning in." You can be "seeing" however not "looking." You can be "hearing" yet not "tuning in."

You are progressively caught up in yourself, in your musings and thoughts, then in the earth outside of you. This condition of central fixation, which is much the same as a fantasy, is a regular or common mesmerizing daze. Another cause of a regular stupor may incorporate being so invested in a book that you are not giving a lot of consideration to what is happening around you. Or on the other hand, you can be caught up in a film, and at some point during that film, you may really get energized or terrified or genuinely engaged with the experience of what you are seeing and hearing. In this season of being so caught up as far as you can tell of wandering off in fantasy land, perusing, viewing a film, or tuning in to music, your considerations—and the sentiments made by your musings—become "genuine," or appear to be at that point. At the point when this occurs, your brain-body or subliminal can't differentiate.

Your pulse may accelerate or back off, muscles may fix or unwind, and you may get ravenous, parched, or queasy. As it were, your brain and body share the experience so well together that it turns into an undeniable physical encounter. Those are regular dazes. As should be obvious, there is no going out, there is no going under. Consistently, you are in charge, and you know that you are in charge. On the off chance that you think about an entrancing stupor similarly as a fantasy, you will have a superior vibe for exactly what it is and what it isn't.

What Hypnosis Is Not

"Hypnosis" may evoke misinterpretations that leave a terrible preference for our mouths. This is expected for the most part to the approach of stage trance. One misinterpretation about hypnosis is that it is "done to" somebody or that an individual "gets mesmerized." This is bogus. Nobody mesmerizes someone else. A decent specialist or clinician just encourages helping individuals figure out how to do this, much as they would figure out how to do contemplation.

Loss of awareness is another misinterpretation. You don't lose awareness when "in a stupor" during hypnosis. Consistently you are completely mindful of where you are and what you are doing. The sleep-inducing stupor itself is like what you experience when you are in a fantasy when you are superbly invested in your contemplations and thoughts. Another misguided judgment about hypnosis is the giving up of your will. Consistently you are in charge and will do nothing without wanting to or your wellbeing.

This incorporates uncovering privileged insights or humiliating yourself. You will do nothing in a stupor that you would not do in a normal waking state. A few people have the bogus thought that they will most likely be unable to come out of stupor. Yet, everybody comes out of daze since they put themselves into it. Hypnosis can normally prompt nodding off, which is a method of coming out of a daze, since rest isn't hypnosis. The distinction among rest and hypnosis is that during rest you are not cognizant. A sleep-inducing daze is a waking state wherein you are caught up in your daydreams and thoughts so completely that you are overlooking the improvements from the earth around you or inside you.

Keep in mind, with hypnosis you are in charge of picking what you need your brain-body to share. You can pick what and how to react. A piece of your body may tingle, however you can decide not to scratch it. The telephone may ring, and you can conclude you don't have to answer it. Getting retained in your considerations and thoughts is the delicate excursion of going into the focal point of yourself that we allude to as "going into a stupor." We may likewise say, "Let yourself dream," or to a kid, we may very well say, "Imagine." Because a dazed state is an aloof or loosened up type of focus or selfabsorption, you will get it going by feeling sufficiently great to allow it to occur.

To be agreeable, you should have a sense of security. That is the reason it is imperative to answer the valid/bogus inquiries concerning what hypnosis truly is and what it truly isn't. Explaining any confusion permits you to see with open-minded perspectives that all that you need is as of now inside you.

The language of Mind-Body

Words are amazing. They are the verbal articulation of musings and thoughts. Your inner mind hears all that you hear, all that you state, and everything that you envision, or imagine. Be that as it may, in particular, your psyche mind deciphers these words and considerations in its language, which isn't exactly a similar language that you intentionally think or talk. Your psyche mind, your brain-body, takes everything.

Intentionally, you think both metaphorically and truly; you can utilize sayings and comprehend what you mean. For instance, you may state, "I need to get thinner so severely." You realize what you mean, however, the inner mind hears something different and reacts to what it hears. For the occasion, let yourself envision the subliminal as a server or server inside your psyche body, taking your request. The exacting comprehension of information disclosed is, "I need to shed pounds ... "

The difference between "trying" and "doing"

We as a whole utilize "try" in our discourse, and we recognize what we mean when we use it. In any case, take a gander at what your inner mind does with "try." Remember, the psyche deciphers everything truly. All in all, what is an "attempt"? We can't see an exacting "attempt," for it is just a metaphor. A "try" doesn't occupy the room or has weight, so it isn't truly there; it is just an idea we use. Attempting to recollect isn't equivalent to recalling. Attempting to nod off isn't equivalent to resting. Attempting to do anything isn't equivalent to doing it, because the result of "endeavoring" can be achievement or disappointment. The psyche interprets "try" into the strict importance of "to try" or "to put being investigated," much like "trying a case" in court. The strict significance is "to see whether." So, the result of "attempt" can be achievement or disappointment, yes or no, valid or bogus. "Doing" is consistently fruitful and can be adjusted by numerous descriptors, for example, quickly, serenely, inadequately, effectively, etc. Notice how the strict message is weakened on the off chance that you put a "try" in the accompanying models: "I am attempting to shed pounds" isn't equivalent to "I am getting in shape." "I am trying to work out" isn't equivalent to "I am accomplishing more exercise." Become touchy to "trying" and instruct yourself to supplant "attempt" with some kind of "do." "I am shedding pounds." "I am going for a stroll in the recreation center tomorrow first thing." Remember the guidance Yoda provided for the youthful warrior Luke in Star Wars: "Do, or don't. There is no try."

Never Is not an option

Émile Coué, a French analyst, composed a book in 1920 about self-hypnosis entitled Self Mastery Through Conscious Autosuggestion. He was maybe the main specialist to advise us that we needn't bother with any other individual to offer us mesmerizing recommendations; we can do it for ourselves. He showed his patients "self-hypnosis" and exhorted them today by day express the words, "Each day, all around, I am improving and better." He likewise prompted, "Never the nots." When talking insistences to yourself, never utilize "not." "not" has no exacting importance to your psyche mind (like "attempt"). You realize what it means, and you use it easily in your cognizant ordinary discourse. Keep in mind, the subliminal just comprehend words on a strict level. For instance, make an effort not to think about a birthday cake. What picture just rung a bell—a pear, a Chevrolet, a giraffe? No, it was presumably an iced cake with lit candles. At the point when you utilize a "not ... something" your psyche mind just hears the "something." Remember Dr. Coue's recommendation, "Never the nots." "I will quit eating when I feel full" rather than "I won't eat excessively." "I will eat one bit of chocolate for dessert" rather than "I won't eat an excess of chocolate." "I will appreciate one serving of potatoes today around evening time" rather than "I won't eat such a large number of potatoes this evening."

The relation between hypnosis and weight loss

At the point when you were a kid, numerous decisions were retained from you, yet now you are a grown-up and have the opportunity to settle on numerous options. Let us take a gander at this thought of how a kid may encounter it. The youngster sees something and needs it, and the sentiment of needing gets overpowering. The kid asks the parent and gets energized with needing the thing wanted. Yet, the youngster can't get it going, because the parent will pick what the parent needs to pick—or possibly that is the way it appears to the kid. Maybe you can recall what it felt like when you truly needed to have something, and it was denied. The kid encounters this refusal as difficult and upsetting. It harms, and the kid may cry or become irate. He may come to accept, "When I am greater, I can have anything I desire." Or the conviction may occur because of being told, "When you are greater, you can pick what you need."

Youngsters don't have the scholarly advancement to comprehend how grown-ups can. The conviction that when they are greater they can have what they need is a type of solace to them. Yet, it is likewise a twofold edged blade, since what does their psyche body (subliminal) do with the words "enormous" and "greater"? It regards them as exacting and cement. "Greater" becomes related to the solace of having the option to have their needs fulfilled and the assurance from that type of passionate torment. Presently, as a grown-up, you realize that the message should signify: "When you are more seasoned and more astute, you can settle on these decisions for yourself." However, the subliminal of the youngster hears "large" and "greater" and deciphers the message actually and with all the passionate vitality present when their needs are being denied. What gets modified into the psyche body? The strict interpretation of "enormous" and "greater" speaks to a major or greater body. Your inner mind doesn't recognize a grown-up body and a major grown-up body—the accentuation is just on "huge." For instance, eight-year-old Annie went out to shop with her mom and a more seasoned sister for Easter dresses. Annie disintegrated in tears when the dress she cherished was not her size. Her more established sister additionally cherished the dress, and it fit her, so her mom got it and told Annie, "When you are greater, you can wear the dress." During a meeting of hypnosis, the grown-up Annie was asked, "Is there any explanation your body needs to clutch abundance weight?" She got upset and tears moved down her cheeks as she reviewed her mom saying, "Annie, you can wear the dress when you are greater." Once this enthusiastic deterrent was uncovered,

Annie had the option to relinquish her abundance weight inside a year. The significant exercise in analyzing these representations and expressions is to consider how the psyche body may act them out genuinely and actually. Keep in mind, your inner mind can't differentiate between what is genuine and what you envision. That is the reason we are welcoming you to mix your creative mind and enjoy your youth specialty of imagining. At the point when you tell your brain-body what you need and what you envision, in the language it comprehends, you will find how that exchange prompts your ideal weight and sound way of life. You will genuinely welcome the grand brain-body association.

How representations can help you in completely changing you

Illustrations are interesting expressions that are valuable to us when speaking with individuals. At the point when we use analogies, we comprehend what we are stating deliberately, however regularly we are not completely mindful of what our psyche body hears. We can't emphasize enough: the psyche body hears words truly and reacts to the exacting importance. We have to disclose to you something extraordinary and essential to recall about your inner mind, the psyche of your body. It can't differentiate between what is genuine and what you envision. This is evident when you consider being inundated in a decent film or novel; our bodies can respond truly to something we envision in the film or novel, similarly as though it were truly occurring. Maybe you have had this experience: You are strolling along a walkway, a path, or even on the floor covering in your home, and you leap off the beaten path of something that ends up being innocuous, a bit of string or an elastic band. In any case, at the time you leaped off the beaten path, there was a piece of you that trusted you should have been leaped off the beaten path, even before you could think to do it. Since your psyche brain couldn't differentiate between what was a genuine or envisioned danger, it bounced you off the beaten path to secure you in either case. Here are a couple of more models: "I simply take a gander at food and put on weight." "Frozen yogurt goes right to my hips." "On the off chance that I stroll past a smorgasbord of pastries, they appear to bounce like magnets to my backside." These are analogies. When individuals offer expressions like these to themselves, to their psyche body, what are they programming their brain-body to do? Is it accurate to say that they are requesting that it hinder their digestion to satisfy the recommendation that seeing food makes them put on weight? Will the psyche body cause them to sweat less, concentrate their pee, hinder the gut motility, or protesting in their stomachs? Keep in mind, it hears words truly and makes every effort to get them going. You may have heard others state, "I can eat anything, and my weight remains the equivalent." If they truly accept that, would they say they are modifying their bodies to do everything to satisfy that conviction and not put on weight? It is safe to say that they are asking the psyche body to accelerate digestion, sweat more, increment their intestinal motility, processing, and end? Will the psyche body make a sentiment of a more prominent feeling of totality much sooner? It hears these words actually, "I can eat anything, and my weight remains the equivalent."

Chapter 3:

The power of guided meditation

Meditation is a natural and effective way of treating psychological problems. Normally people use meditation to improve their inner self as it helps in increasing the person's concentration and keeps him alert and focus in his daily routine life. Meditation is an easy way to remove all the toxic emotions from the mind such as anger, fear, stress, excessive worry, lack of concentration, depression, and many others. A more refined and advanced form of meditation is known as guided mediation which can be used to attain inner stillness and can help you to enter into a deep state of relaxation. Guided mediation is a powerful tool to eliminate stress and as a result, positive personal changes start showing up. Guided meditation is also known as guided imagery meditation.

Guided meditation is performed under the supervisor of a meditation teacher, or through listening to a recording or specific mediation music. Meditation guides will instruct you either to sit calmly or may ask you to lie down depending upon your physical condition. After following the basic instructions regarding the posture, your guide will start talking to you and ask you to concentrate on his words. These words of your mediator will lead you to the world of relaxing visualizations. You will then start feeling the relaxing vibes and gradually your stress starts getting fade away. At this point your mind becomes clear and your way of analyzing things becomes different. You will start taking things lightly and positively. This is the point when your guide will take you to an inner journey which can help you in discovering various aspects of your life. If you are performing guided meditation for a specific purpose then you have to mention it to your mediator. Guided meditation can be used for various purposes like for empowering personal positive thinking, emotional healing, spiritual development, weight loss, to unleash your full potential, to get the pleasure of deep relaxation, increasing alertness or focus, or for overcoming stress and depression.

Relationship of guided meditation with weight loss
Your body is your icon and people normally recognize you through your body. Whenever your name comes to their mind, your whole image appears. Having a smart and sleek body attracts everyone and personally speaking I love to have a good athletic body. I use various natural and effective methods to maintain the standards of ideal body shape. According to my personal experience, guided meditation is one of the easiest and effective methods to get an ideal body. One of the major cause of body fat or D-shaped body is excessive stress and depression. People who normally thinks a lot and

perform less physical activity starts getting fat. This particular problem has nothing to do with excessive eating because most people believe that eating is the major cause of obesity. If you want to overcome the problem of your body fat then you have to eliminate the basic reason which is stress.

Most people start using prescription drugs to overcome anxiety and stress which causes obesity but according to my experience avoid medication as it mostly causes side effects. Try to adopt those measures which can help in achieving your desired results without effecting your body. Meditation is a helpful way of overcoming the problem of stress which will ultimately lead you towards achieving your desired body. In the process of guided meditation, you undergo the process of developing a strong will of attaining your specified goals. Guided mediation helps in making your mind strong so that you can achieve your targets.

Guided meditation is not only restricted to attain relaxation. It is a method to upgrade yourself and transform your way of thinking into an entirely new dimension of positivity and growth. Guided meditation is an effortless and enjoyable experience of attaining immense relaxation, detoxing negative emotions, and achieving the positive aspects of life. When it comes to weight loss, you have to mention this specifically to your mediator guide. He will help you in getting into the specific state of mind which controls obesity and boosts your will to fight your excessive will of eating. Once you have mastered the eating requirements of your body then you can easily control your diet. This is an easy and effective way to overcome obesity.

Once your session of guided meditation ends, your guide will gradually bring you back to the normal state of awareness. After completing the session of guided meditation, you will start feeling relaxed, refreshed, and rejuvenated. The duration of guided meditation varies from 5 minutes to 60 minutes depending on your requirement. Normally, a session of 20 minutes or longer is advised to people. This is an ideal duration to attain a deep state of relaxation which can maximize the positive benefits of meditation.

Difference between Guided Mediation and Traditional Meditations

In traditional meditation techniques, you take your concentration on a single point of focus without having any external support or guide. Single point of focus in traditional meditation can be a specific physical action, to maintain a focus on your breathing, or it can be a mantra or a sound, a word or phrase which you have to repeat to yourself mentally. These simple meditation techniques are effective in attaining inner peace and stillness. After completing a few sessions of your meditation, you will observe that your ability to concentrate is also enhanced. Some people find it difficult to meditate on their own. For them, it is better to learn effective ways of meditation from experts or adopt guided meditation.

Most people go for guided meditation because it doesn't require any previous training and expertise. Even if you are an extremely stressed person and finds it difficult to overcome your thoughts than guided mediation can help you in easing your pressure. With the help of guided meditation, you can easily attain a deep state of inner relaxation and peace of mind. Your guide will take you into the deep state of your inner self which can help in discovering the hidden potential. This is the best way to dig out the positivity of yourself. This type of meditation is mostly recommended for people who are new to meditation or want to learn meditation. People who are well experienced in performing meditation can also get the benefit of guided meditation. Guided imagery meditations are mostly used by experienced meditators to take the person into a deeper and vivid state of mediation. This deeper state of relaxation can help the person in attaining specific goals which are normally not possible in traditional meditation. Guided meditation is different from traditional meditation as it uses music or any other natural sound to enhance the experience of meditation.

Role of Music in guided imagery meditation

Tranquil meditation music is mostly used in guided imagery meditation. This music and sounds will help you in getting relaxed during the session of guided meditations. Just imagine how a simply a good soundtrack in a movie makes it more interesting and enjoyable. Guided meditation follows the same principle and delivers the benefits of meditation through music. With the help of soothing music, your mind can take a journey into the deep dimensions of your mind where you can attain the feelings of deep relaxation. Concentrating on the music will fly you away from the stressful thoughts of your mind.

For guided meditation, specific CD's and MP3's are also available which includes the sounds of nature and other soothing music. All these sounds are quite relaxing which can be used to enhance the vividness of visualizations. For example, if you are guided to visualize yourself standing in a lush green forest, then your experience of that visualization will be more authentic if you hear the sound birds. Another example of a guided visualization is when you are guided to visualize yourself standing on a sandy beach. Your visualization becomes more authentic when you hear the sound of ocean waves.

In traditional meditation, the main focus of the person is to attain mental stillness through concentration exercises. On the other hand, guided meditation follows the principle of strong and vivid series of visualizations, music and natural environmental sounds to increase your attention, to relax you, and to take you to an inner journey. Guided meditation is mostly aimed to achieve specific outcomes that are why guided meditation is a more powerful tool than traditional meditation. Guided mediation is a helpful tool in developing your mental and physical skills. People who are suffering from the problem of obesity or simply want to maintain their weight and body shape can use a guided meditation. I am using the techniques of guided meditation for years to maintain my body weight. It is a preventive and effective way to overcome the problem of body weight. Your body is your temple which represents you. You have to spend all your time with your body. So, everyone must take proper care of their bodies. Meditation is one of the best ways to fight mental and physical problems together at the same time.

Why People need guided meditation

Individuals who practice guided meditation are intense lovers, who need to relax, or those who are achieving self-awareness and or want to get any specific goal. It is mostly used by beginners who have no prior experience of mediation and require guidance for learning the techniques of meditation. It is perfect for individuals who are looking for a relaxed and stress-free life, or those needing to be happier and healthier in life.

Guided meditation (which is also known as guided relaxation) is mostly applied for relaxing purposes, for emotional and physical healing and also for spiritual development. It is a proven method to loosen up the mind and accomplish inner peace. The purpose of guided meditation is to assist you in the direction where you lose your connection with the outside world, freeing your mind from all kinds of worries and stress, through following the expression and words of your guide. Various individuals have confidence in the viability of guided meditation and declare it as the best technique for relaxing and getting inner peace. The best thing about guided meditation is that it has no side-effects and applies to people of all ages.

Meditation is an effective and easy way to discharge all the negative thoughts and energy stored in your body. With the help of deep relaxation techniques, you can reach the hidden parts of your mind or can travel through those relaxing thoughts which were hidden in the lost compartments of your mind. Due to excessive stress and workload pressure, positive thoughts and joyful memories normally fade away. This experience can release the intensity of the inner mind to discharge positive thinking. Keep in mind, our mind and thinking process resembles a computer that can be customized according to our needs and requirements. If you need to change your perspective to turn out to be increasingly profitable in any part of your life, guided meditation can be an answer. There are a few guided meditation procedures that will suit your necessities.

No one can measure the level of success which is attained through guided meditation. Guided meditation is a method of self-healing and relaxation. Relaxing or meditation is frequently done with soothing music, with sounds of nature, or through combing both. It includes deep breathing techniques and vivid visualizations that can relax the brain. Individuals who utilize guided meditation regularly find inner joy and calmness throughout everyday life. Guided meditation is an effective treatment method for those people who are suffering from extreme stress and anxiety disorder. The emotional wellbeing and psychological health of an individual plays an important role in his daily activities. A regular session of guided meditation can protect a person from different kinds of psychological issues.

Techniques of Guided Meditation

Normally, the mind is the major hurdle while doing meditation. The mind plays different techniques to spoil the essence of mediation and tries to keep the person in a constant state of depression and anxiety. Sometimes the mind appears to be a different entity that is performing against the will of the person.

In any case, never forget the true purpose of your mind which is to serve its master and that is you. Always remember that a mind is only a tool that can be used to perform tasks. The mind is also used as a pathway for meditation. Among the various techniques of meditation, an effective technique is known as guided meditation. Guided meditation is normally performed at the end of your regular yoga class.

A human mind is a powerful tool that can lead you to the world of imagination. That is why guided medication depends upon the mind and to get the best results from a guided medication you have to use your mind effectively. The individual imagines predefined situations as defined by the guide will take you into the world of imagination. Since the eyes are closed in guided meditation, the recommended visualization should either be from memory or listened through a guide or audio. Reading is not an option in a guided meditation.

One may record themselves in advance and listen to it during the process of mediation or they may approach a friend to read the lines while you are meditating because some people may find it distracting to listen to their voice during meditation. There is no hard rule for guided mediation but try to choose a method that suits you perfectly.

The human mind can be differentiated into two major states known as the conscious mind and the unconscious mind. The unconscious mind can't differentiate between reality and fiction. Whatever the unconscious mind sees it believes it as truth. This is the reason why some people feel terrified while watching a horror movie or they start crying after witnessing a tragic scene. On the other hand, the conscious mind realizes that a film isn't real, but the unconscious mind believes it real. For that degree of the mind, it happened. The same thing can be said for our thoughts and imaginations. The things we often dream in our mind mostly impacts our physical life. At the point when we undergo stressful situations, our pulse goes up, the palms begin sweating, and the process of breathing becomes difficult.

This crucial part of the brain is normally utilized passively and never deliberately, which is a total waste of potential powers of the mind. With guided meditation, the unconscious mind is converted into a powerful tool to attain inner peace.

Peaceful surrounding environment and comfort should be maintained properly before entering into the process of guided meditation. Wear loose and comfortable clothes and get the body into a place where it can stay for a longer period without feeling any pain. Get settled in the desired position and afterward hold up for a moment or two. In case more movement or adjustment is required do that now. When up think that you have settled completely than start your meditation.

There is a wide range of guided meditation options available out there. You can choose one according to your need and requirement which suits you perfectly. Pure light guided meditation involves distinctively imagining light surroundings and being indulged in your own body completely. This is a method of purifying and cleaning all the impurities from the body and helps the person in healing all kinds of emotional wounds. Another type of guided meditation is imagining oneself as a tree, visualizing your body as the bark of the trees whose roots are going into the ground. This technique is known as grounding meditation. There are several other guided meditation techniques and each has its effects. You have to ascertain your need first before choosing any type of guided meditation.

Effective Guided Meditation

Guided meditation is one of the simplest ways of relaxation. It is a proven method to ease the pressure of the mind and to eliminate all the negative energy from the body. In this method of relaxation, you have to adjust your body in a relaxing pose which can be either sitting on a chair or laying on your back. Choose a position that is easy to maintain and comfortable. You may find some difficulty in the beginning sessions of your meditation but after completing a few successful sessions of meditation, you will become an expert. After becoming an expert in meditation you will learn how to control your emotions, feelings which will ultimately lead you to inner peace.

No matter which method you adopt to perform guided meditation, all have their own benefits. Here are a few techniques that can be used in a guided meditation to get its maximum benefit.

The first step in effective guided meditation is to choose a comfortable position which can help in getting relaxed easily. There is no particular position; you could either sit, lean back on a chair seat, or even sit with folded legs on a bed. You simply have to be comfortable and easy. Try to avoid those postures which can cause pain at the end of your meditation session.

Next, you need to get relax. Try to take deep breathes and maintain your heartbeat for relaxing purposes. Another approach for relaxing is to close your eyes and focus on your anxieties. At that point, the center on these burdens and try to constrain them out.

After getting the vibes of calmness and relaxation, now you have to move to the next step. Close your eyes and imagine your spirit moving out of your body and skimming over your head. The whole purpose of meditation is to build-up for this specific moment. Nobody can directly reach this point without following the initial steps. When you feel that your spirit is flying away, try to make trips to those places which can help you in getting relaxed. Most people feel relaxed at the sandy beaches, most people like green forests, and some people like mountains. Whatever destination you like, keep your focus on that particular point until your mind gets completely calmed and relaxed. In guided meditation music or nature, sounds play a vital role in taking you to the depths of calmness.

Guided meditation is all about understanding your own body and mind. The relaxing environment and meditation both are different things according to some people who perform meditation regularly. Some would imagine themselves on a tropical island with remarkable scenes, while others would like to imagine themselves in the forested areas among blossoms and trees. No matter which place you like for relaxation but the main purpose of meditation is to consider yourself in those beautiful locations during the process of guided meditation.

Guided meditation is all about your imagining power and the power of visualization. You have to stay in your imaginary world until you start feeling relaxed and calm. Try to take all your senses with you while you are meditating. See and feel the beauty of the scene, smell the fragrance of flowers, and appreciate the sounds of flying birds and running water. After completing the session of your meditation, feel the lightness of your soul while traveling back from the beautiful environment and entering back into your body. At the point when you are back, you will feel refreshed and relaxed. You will get the same feelings as you get while returning from short vacations. When performing guided meditation, you can use some soothing music that can help you to get relax in no time.

Guided Meditation is all about training and practice. Each time you perform guided meditation, try to gradually increase your time in your imaginary environment. Additionally, with training, guided meditation will have positive and powerful effects on the people who are suffering from extreme pressure issues.

According to mind studies, the human brain acts and operates according to the body. As your body reacts to the situation, it has a direct impact on the brain. When a person goes through a stressful situation all the good energy from the body is drained out. In these scenarios, specialists have suggested that, with the help of guided meditation, the brain can regain the positive energy back which can be then distributed to the body. Meditation and guided meditation requires some patience and self-control. After mastering the techniques of mediation, you can learn how to control your emotions, feelings, overcome stress, and heal your broken thoughts. The outcome of guided meditation is quick and positive. Individuals of all ages can practice this type of therapy to overcome their physical and psychological issues.

The basic reason for meditation is to get your physical body to align with your mind so that both can operate in harmony. When this synchronization happens, your ability to respond to the daily stress increases significantly. Now you can effectively operate in any kind of situation and can easily bear huge workload pressure through overcoming your stress. Although this sounds unrealistic, it isn't. The power of meditation is quite astonishing.

With regular training and practice, guided meditation will help you to discover your hidden powers and shows you the real capabilities of your mind. Always believe in yourself and keep making positive changes in your personality. This is a key component when you want to change your thought process to make yourself a better person for society. Make yourself believe that great changes will occur. Guided meditation is an excellent healing process when performed regularly. This will ease the weight of stress and pressure from your mind and body.

Using guided meditation for weight loss

In case you love eating and mostly eat more than others than it can create problems in your body and you will find it difficult to perform your daily tasks. Most bad eating habits are developed after witnessing stressful events in life. You may think that you can control your diet but whenever any stressful event hits your life again, you will start eating more. This problem cannot be solved temporarily and needs some permanent solution.

For compulsive eaters, guided meditation is the best solution for their problem. It allows them to eat mindfully rather than eating mindlessly. There is a big difference between eating with mind and eating without mind. Eating food while sitting in front of the TV while giving no consideration to the taste or texture of the food and eating food as fast as possible are two examples of mindless eating. Such activities mostly lead to overeating or eating carelessly without giving you any idea about when to stop. You urge to eat more remains in your mind as you have enjoyed no taste of your food. This will lead you to excessive eating which can result in taking more calories each day.

On the other hand, when you eat with an attentive mind you focus on all the details of the food you are eating like witnessing the flavor and texture of every single bite you bring. The pace of eating with an open mind is slow rather than eating with mindlessly. Eating in this manner will allow you to take more time which will help your digestion system to work properly. In this way, you will feel full in less time which will result in taking fewer calories. Sometimes your stomach takes 20 minutes to send the signal to the brain about the when to stop eating. By eating an appropriate amount of food each day, you will take fewer calories in your body which will lead you toward weight loss.

Guided meditation is the best way to train your mind about specific things. The main purpose of guided meditation is to overcome stress-related issues, healing emotional problems, and training the body and mind to work together. Once your mind is trained, you can easily control your mind according to your will. With the help of guided meditation, you can discover the hidden potential of your mind and can attain inner peace.

Chapter 4:

The Power Of Affirmations

You need to know that affirmations are one of the most powerful things that we are blessed with. With affirmations, there is nothing that you cannot achieve. I realized the power of affirmations when I started applying them in my own life. An affirmation is defined by many researchers and philosophers. A simple definition of an affirmation is the continuously repeated expression of a wish. Affirmations are consciously chosen by a person and in this chapter, we will dwell deep in this topic and help you understand how they can help you in changing your overall life.

The universe is energy. It follows the laws of nature. The same is the case with the thoughts. Thoughts are creative. You need to know that you have access to unlimited energy and you only need to find a way to tap into it and unlock all the mysteries. The mysteries of the body can be unlocked with the help of a streamlines thought process. You need to know that thoughts are a form of energy and energy does not wander away in nothingness. Thoughts have an impact on your life and the lives of the people around you. We are thinking all the time and it takes a lot of practice to empty your mind. Believe me, you will not be able to spend a few minutes without thinking anything. People tend to ignore the thoughts, they do not know whether they are thinking positive or negative. Thoughts have value and they work in different ways. The power of affirmations can be felt individually and collectively.

Thoughts and Subconscious

We have a consciousness, which permits us to think, however, we likewise have a subliminal where all contemplations are being spared. It has a trustworthy memory and it acknowledges what it is told without dissenting. It controls the elements of our bodies, yet additionally our activities. When there is a contention between our will and our psyche, the last wins. Much the same as a PC our psyche has a specific sparing example. Comparative musings which are being thought, communicated, or recorded will – when rehashed - become fixed in our psyche, which is in certainty our hard plate. From that point, they act self-governing, in any event, when we don't know about this. They follow up on our condition since the other unwittingly get these considerations and act as per them, except if they need to acknowledge different things through their own picked contemplations.

Daydreams of a specific topic, a specific occasion, a specific feeling will draw in one another and will wrap up. That makes them more grounded and they can act better on what they speak to. When there are numerous musings about a similar subject, these become thought around that subject framing a bad-to-the-bone. This center can be taken care of with numerous or just negative musings or by numerous or just positive considerations or by 9 contemplations of the two sorts. Regardless of whether it is a positive or a negative center along these lines relies upon which sort of contemplations wins.

At the point when it is a negative center and when it increased a fixed structure, it will begin to draw in its reciprocals, this implies the negative things coordinated in it. The equivalent occurs with a positive center. As a center of considerations is being framed, it turns out to be increasingly ground-breaking and ready to acknowledge obviously and immovably what it speaks to, as per the idea with which it was constructed. All musings that were once spared stay there until we choose to eradicate them and that is the reason they can be seen by others. Musings consistently emerge, remember that, except if we purposefully choose to transform them.

Two Fundamental Thoughts

There are in reality just two principal considerations: dread and love. The various contemplations can be followed back to those two considerations. It tends to be very light up to find the genuine beginning of our and others' contemplations. At the point when the crucial idea is dread for what it's worth for envy, outrage, hatred, pomposity, and so on and when we perceive this essential idea in another person, this encourages us to understand that the other one in actuality just communicates his apprehensions and that for example, his upheaval of outrage depends on the dread of not having (not having love), not being (not being adored) and that it isn't outraged thusly.

At the point when we are apprehensive, there is no adoration at that point and the other way around. Dread can't be prohibited by dread, however by a caring methodology. Cherishing in the broadest feeling of the word, since it is difficult to request that we love somebody we don't adore. Anyway, it is at that point conceivable to attempt to accomplish a circumstance of rest, for example by sending the idea: "I wish you concordance and health in any region". When even that is excessively, and this is conceivable, one would then be able to send an idea, for example, "I favor you and set you free" or still "We leave each other's lives incongruity or we are both free".

Love is more significant than fear as the number of vibrations is higher. We can decide on it whenever it is our decision. Subsequently, contemplations borne by adoration have a more grounded intensity of acknowledgment. These considerations relate to the reality of our reality. They offer assurance.

How to phrase affirmations

This is a significant thing. You should initially choose what you need precisely. Not what another person wishes, no trade-off between existing circumstances, however what you wish, somewhere down in your heart. At the point when you have questions, when your desire is unclear, keep on contemplating it until you make certain about what you truly need and about the – in any event a base - of the plausibility of it. At that point, the expression of your attestation will be all the more persuasive. You can likewise figure out what you need rather than what you have thus characterized an undesirable circumstance, which you would then be able to change in its inverse, in particular a needed circumstance.

It very well may be for example, that you believe you are being disregarded in your relationship because your accomplice doesn't consider what you need. You would then be able to characterize unequivocally what it is and record the contrary idea, something you do need. Allude additionally to the section on "basic examples". You can reach skyward, even high, however, your desire ought to stay practical, not something of which you are very certain that it is difficult to figure it out. All in all, you can set up whether it is a genuine wish for you. Still, you need to attempt to find whether this desire is of any utilization for your self-awareness. The desire can be arranged in any territory. You don't need to be reluctant to wish something arranged in the material territory. Try not to discuss what this desire could be accurate except if that individual wants you to enjoy all that life has to offer and has an extremely inspirational mentality (that implies that you infrequently can discuss your desires before their acknowledgment).

Wishes can at times be utilized as a spread to escape a specific circumstance or they can shroud an absence of adoration or be remuneration for something that you don't have and that would 15 be able to be increasingly central. You must consider this stage. Try not to fear what you may find and of the genuine issue. Envision that you have achieved your desire: does this fulfill you? Does it cause you to feel great? Is the thought process behind it great? Is it something that is yours?

We should respond to the inquiry in the case of something that feels bravo, just for us and we are the main ones that can offer a response. Regardless of whether target specialists as of now have offered us a response. There is no total aptitude in the field of others' desires. Nothing is incomprehensible on the off chance that it feels bravo. Try not to request something that isn't explicit: if you wish to have more riches, at that point don't request a generously compensated activity, however, request what you genuinely need. On the off chance that you need to travel, don't request the cash to go out traveling, however concerning the outing itself. It may be the case that regardless of whether your desire for cash has emerged, a wide range of obstructions keep you from making the excursion.

While communicating your desire overlook for once absolutely that one must be benevolent, that you don't reserve the option to wish solely what you need. Try not to consider the desires of others. Simply consider the accompanying significant condition that your desire must not hurt anybody to any degree. Therefore you don't need to solicit the authorization from another person, don't get some information about it, just get some information about it. Your most profound self. You know for certain what can be hurtful for other people, so you are totally capable, in all receptiveness, to figure out what you can "defend" by methods for assertions.

Killing Negative Thoughts

When pondering what it is you truly need and recording it to make the confirmation structure, it tends to be that you record something that conflicts with your sentiments. At the point when a desire doesn't feel right, at that point leave it.

Emotions are a generally excellent standard to decide if a desire is beneficial for you or not. Thinking alone isn't adequate, because you 16 need to connect it to the inclination you need to understand your desire as quickly as time permits. So you must be glad when you see what you have recorded. So cheerful that you yell with satisfaction when you picture that your desire will be achieved. At the point when this is the situation, at that point it is okay.

Emotions are additionally a decent standard to quantify the vitality of a confirmation. At the point when you wish to be thin and utilize the confirmation: "I am presently thin" while you are glancing despondently in the mirror believing that you are not thin by any stretch of the imagination, that will cause you to feel awful while communicating your attestation.

The vitality to emerge the attestation won't be extremely high or even negative, at the end of the day it could even give you a greater amount of what you don't need. This is because your conviction overcomes. That is the reason it is imperative to divert when you are not feeling so great, either by dispensing with the fundamental examples, the pessimistic feelings, either by convincing and persuading yourself regarding the way that what you wish has just become genuine so often for others, by envisioning your certification and potentially by making a file card

During the time spent recording it can happen that you are communicating your desire, yet that at that point the accompanying considerations spring up:

- Do I merit this?

- Is it practical?

- I need more ability for that

- I am unreasonably old for that

- I need more an ideal opportunity for that

- Shall I despise everything be cherished when I have this or when I am that?

- Won't I lose it immediately? Etc.

Daydreams happening to you when expressing your desire are associated with how you see things. Conceivably without you staying alert about it. They show you the point you have to "chip away at". These internal protections are acceptable gauges to find out about how you feel about yourself, your self-regard.

Dispensing with those protections is a procedure that might be a higher priority than emerging your desire.

They give you what you have to tidy up on your approach to building up your desire, at the end of the day, yourself. As we have seen previously, your desire is a piece of you. It is the manual for the more complete individual you can turn into. The flawlessness inside your compass. Else, I need to rehash it, you could never have that craving. It would not have been put inside you. Wishes are not discretionarily placed into somebody's heart, however just on the off chance that they are intended for that particular heart. The most effective method to do the tidying up? Composing an assertion communicating something contrary to the "prospect of obstruction". For example when you have questions about whether you merit it: "I merit (for example to be love or to acquire X Euros)".

Or on the other hand when you wonder whether you can even now do this on your age: "Age doesn't make a difference, presently is the correct second. Or then again to eradicate a sentiment of vulnerability: "I generally feel quiet and quiet". At the point when such an attestation incites another idea of obstruction, in for example the model referenced above "I generally feel quiet and quiet" and you abruptly think "aside from when X says something explicit or when he blows up", you need to change this into something positive for yourself: "I feel tranquil and quiet likewise when X says either". In this way, toward the starting, you can, alongside the new and picked attestation, likewise record something contrary to the feelings ruining the achievement of your desire. Perhaps you can put directly inverse one another.

This may prompt another "tidying up process". So leave enough spot to record new feelings of dread or feelings. At that point, you need to make new confirmations communicating something contrary to these feelings of trepidation, feelings, negative contemplations. These "incited" confirmations must be made until these contrary daydreams quit bouncing up. So you no longer substitute the method of your desire. Basic examples of musings can be exceptionally profound.

It's a given that when you are communicating a confirmation without considerations of opposition happening, you can go on with it. At that point you need to feel that what is in your certification can turn out to be valid, considerably more, as of now is valid for you, and as we have seen before it significant that you feel great while communicating your desire. In that manner, you can truly have confidence in it. So in the theory referenced over, the uncertainty or incredulity emerging is a reflection of what is in our inner mind.

Uncertainty dependent on an absence of has confidence in one's prospects, because of circumstances previously or too contrasting oneself as well as other people as opposed to reacting to your one of a kind self. So tune in to your interesting being, shaped by your one of a kind capacities and abilities, by the totally one of a kind type of vitality of it. So when your inner mind "fights" when you express a desire, stating the assertion isn't sufficient. All things considered, we are consistently the total of all considerations spared sooner or later and these keep on creating their belongings. Thus, there ought not to be any logical inconsistency between what you state as a desire and what you think may occur. All things considered, you don't accept emphatically enough and it could have a contrary impact.

As we have seen previously, inverse feelings kill one another and the most grounded conviction consistently wins. Then again, questions which are in reality the rebelliousness among cognizance and subliminal can have a contrary impact too, which is in actuality by what we said in the past segment. It tends to be that what you feel, that your inner mind, your instinct discloses to you that it is best not to accept that new position, however another. Still, you have questions since you consider notoriety, compensation, and so on.

Your cognizant psyche reveals to you that it is not sensible not to pick the generously compensated activity as from the target perspective, that activity will give you numerous points of interest. At the point when you don't pick the activity as per your emotions and instincts because your explanation discloses to you that the other one is greatly improved, this would do your profound wish a lot of wrongs. It is likewise a reality, regardless of whether that seems unimaginable at that point, that permitting that unbelievable chance to pass, may make opportunities for a surprisingly better deal. You stay consistent with yourself. You being aware of that permits you to understand your desires quicker.

Why Use Affirmations?

Is this extremely valuable? Wishes are placed into us because their emergence is beneficial for us since they cause us to feel great, improve our turn of events, make us move along. Wishes cause us to feel alive. As we have said previously, a precarious issue is to know whether our desires are our actual wishes and not enlivened by dread or comparative sentiments. Look at the thought process of your desire. Learning the assertion method causes us to hold the condition of bliss, to make us less vulnerable to evolving states of mind. Certifications can be utilized to feel increasingly peaceful, to have the option to see solidarity with others. Each progression is forever procured. On account of this strategy, you have the way to adapt to a wide range of circumstances that initially seemed, by all accounts, to be impossible.

Assertions can fix what has been pounded into our subliminal for quite a long time by negative contemplations, without us monitoring it. Try not to be amazed or frantic when a confirmation doesn't in a flash become valid. It initially needs to confront and delete all the negative things in our psyche obstructing the acknowledgment of the certification. Moreover, there can be a ton of hindrances around us, of which we have no clue. Having confidence that everything is to our benefit is an essential fundamental demeanor. 33 Affirmations can square undesirable aims: "I am in any capacity shielded from harming impacts of others". This can be helpful to shield us from individuals taking our vitality, generally unwittingly, which happens more frequently than one may might suspect.

What's to come is controlled by our present musings, which are as we have said previously, installed in our atmosphere. At the point when our example of musings keeps on being equal, we can distinguish a future occasion dependent on how we have made it. This implies we can change our future whenever by changing our musings. Nothings stay steady, nothing deteriorates, everything is continually developing.

The inquiry of whether our total course of life can be changed, as it were its amount is foreordained, is one of the most troublesome issues. It appears to me that everything is a consequence voluntarily. A decision to emerge a desire or a decision not to appear it, a decision not to accept that it is conceivable. It is because of the absence of conviction that undesired conditions in life happen. Such conditions are regularly alluded to as "it is my fate". Attestations saying that "it generally transpires, I am consistently the person in question, and so forth." emerge a self-made supposed "fate", which can whenever be changed. Is there a general parcel, a fate? As in no desire can be placed into us without us having the option to appear it, which additionally implies that the ability to do so is available and simultaneously as in no desire is the equivalent, that everybody communicates it remarkably, that he in actuality needs to do one or the other wishes never can be conflicting concerning both the singularity and the collectivity of people, there is the fate that desires orchestrate with one another. This implies the wish is useful for us all.

Withdrawing from this fundamental guideline implies that the desire will appear such that meets the antiquated standards of agreement, harmony, happiness, and cooperative attitude. If not, there will be disorder and a wide range of negative conditions, including questions. The total apparatus depends on one actuality that was given to our awareness. The opportunity of thought. We can't change the law that contemplations become things, however, we can utilize it. Openly. Continuously openly, for right and wrong. Anyway, it isn't generally important to realize how everything functions, it is even not important to realize that it works. Without singular decisions from one viewpoint, the collectivity of musings on the other, the various circumstances wherein people are living, are conceived, pass on, would not happen.

Would one be able to contend that, when one is curious about with the intensity of contemplations, he is compelled to come or to calmly acknowledge the acknowledgment of his desires or the cynicism on the planet? Furthermore, he isn't the reason for existence with our without complete self-acknowledgment? We can just answer this by saying that likewise, obliviousness has its belongings. Likewise, numbness is a decision. Albeit presently this is being tended to an ever-increasing extent. What it is about is that everybody is the main cognizant mastermind in their life on the off chance that the person needs it and that the individual can go past the undesirable conditions.

History gives us numerous models. Individuals have figured out how to go from unpleasant neediness, both material and profound, to extraordinary riches, additionally both material and otherworldly, by acknowledging incredible achievements and developments, by becoming extraordinary pioneers, be getting extraordinary riches, by the entirety of that simultaneously. At the point when we need another future, it is critical to quit focusing on the past. I rehash that by focusing our consideration on something, we fortify it.

We can use for example the accompanying confirmation for this: "The past doesn't longer exist. Starting now and into the foreseeable future, I make a present and a future as I need them to be". It is likewise significant that we understand that every day is a fresh start. An everlasting chance to begin once more. We don't need to convey the heap of past encounters. We have the ability to delete them when we don't need them to be a piece of us. Your "part" is in certainty your psychological demeanor: the manner in which you feel, accept and think will form your future.

Chapter 5: How to Use Meditation and Affirmations to Lose Weight

You have learned about the power of meditation and affirmations in the previous chapter. Whether you are planning to lose weight or bring positivity in your life, affirmations and meditations are some of the best tools you can have. We will discuss how the body works and how the mind-body connection and energy psychology can help you lose weight.

You control the essential ingredients that make meditation work for you. These are the same ingredients that create your experience of success for any goal you choose. Let us look at each element and how you may use it to perform for you.

Motivation
Motivation is the vitality of your longing, of what you need. Needing is an inclination that you can control. For a large portion of your life, you have essentially controlled your longing or needing by restricting it or denying it. You might be truly adept at controlling your wants and needing in certain zones and frail or fresh in others. Since this is a "diet" book, you may have just set yourself up to hear that this "diet" will resemble the others and I will showcase the points which you can accept or deny. Having a good diet is essential but staying motivated is equally imperative. That is,

different weight control plans have mentioned to you what you need, and the accentuation may have been about "not needing" a few nourishments that you have developed to adore. Welcome to another method of rewarding yourself; I will urge you to show signs of improvement at "needing." Denial is excluded from The Self-Hypnosis Diet.

Your motivation is a key factor, one of the basic fixings. We need you to center your vitality of needing not toward food yet toward the inspiration that tells your mind-body what you need it to make: immaculate weight. I urge you to get great at needing your ideal weight. Here is a model. Let us state that you are in a pool, and out of nowhere you take in a significant piece of water. At that time, you need just a single thing, a breath of air. It feels desperate, and a breath of air is the main thing at the forefront of your thoughts as of now. The needing is so serious and ground-breaking that it eclipses every single other idea and impels you to take the necessary steps to get that breath of air. That is the amount we need you to need the weight and self-perception that you want.

Belief
Beliefs are those thoughts that are valid for you. They don't need to be experimentally demonstrated for you to realize that they generally will be valid for you. Regardless of whether you know about it or not, your activities, both cognizant and subliminal, depend on

your convictions and beliefs. Although your beliefs are as thoughts, they shape your experience by influencing your activities throughout everyday life. If you accept that espresso keeps you conscious around evening time, you presumably don't drink espresso before heading to sleep. The intensity of accepting lets you impact your body in manners that may appear to be shocking.

On the off chance that an individual truly accepts that he will get well when taking specific medicine, it will happen whether the tablet contains a prescription or is just latent. Similarly, if an individual truly accepts that he can accomplish high evaluations in school, it will occur. When an individual truly accepts that he can achieve his ideal weight, it will occur.

Recall your games as a youngster. Your capacity to imagine is similarly as solid now as when you were youthful. It might be somewhat corroded, and you may require a touch of training, however when you permit yourself to imagine and let yourself trust in what you are imagining, you will find an integral asset. You will find this is a brilliantly successful approach to convey your goals, those messages of what you need, to the entirety of the phones and tissues and organs of your body, which react by bringing that aim into reality for you. We can't state this enough: considerations are things. The considerations, the photos, the thoughts you put in your brain become the messages your self-hypnosis passes on to your mind-body, at last transforming your ideal body into a reality. Imagining is picking what to accept and getting ingested in those thoughts. Similarly, as an amplifying glass can center beams of daylight, you can center your psychological vitality to make your musings, thoughts, and convictions genuine for your body.

Expectations

You may not generally get what you need, yet you do get what you anticipate. Desires contain the vitality of convictions and become the aftereffects of what is accepted. Here is a case of how to "anticipate." When you plunked down to peruse this book, you didn't look at the seat or couch to test its capacity to hold your weight. You just plunked down without pondering it. You didn't need to consider it, because a piece of you is sure, and has such a great amount of confidence in the seat, that you simply "anticipated" it to hold you. That is how to expect the ideal body weight you want. Remembering this, be aware of what you state to yourself as well as other people concerning your body weight desires. "I generally put on weight over the special seasons." "The previous evening I ate two bits of cake, and early today I was two pounds heavier."

Meditation for perfect mind and body

Every one of the fundamental ingredients can create ground-breaking results when centered inside the brain-body. Nonetheless, when these ingredients are adjusted appropriately inside the procedure of self-hypnosis, their adequacy has amplified a hundredfold.

Self-hypnosis is a procedure for making your world. You may think this sounds mystical or unrealistic, however, that is comparative with what you have encountered so far in your life. These thoughts might be extremely new to you. Here is a case of the "relative" nature of new thoughts. Envision that you are given a personal jet that is wonderfully furnished with lavish arrangements and an all-around prepared team. It is a superb blessing, and you get the chance to show this building wonder to certain people who have seen nothing like it.

To state that self-hypnosis is a procedure by which you make your existence may appear to be unrealistic or even extraordinary at the present time, possibly as phenomenal as a time machine is for a few. That is fine, for the present moment; however open your mind and creative mind to the conceivable outcomes that this offers you to accomplish your ideal body weight. Let yourself accept that this procedure is genuine and valid, because it is, and because it depends upon your conviction to turn out to be valid. Your inner (mind-body) utilizes the mix of what you need (inspiration), what you accept, and what you expect as an outline for activity. The outcomes are accomplished by your brain-body (subliminal), and not by intuition or breaking down.

If an individual contact a virus surface that she accepts is extremely hot, she can deliver a rankle or consume reaction. On the other hand, an individual contacting an extremely hot surface reasoning that it is cool may not create a consume reaction. Individuals who stroll over hot coals while envisioning that they are cool may encounter a warm physical issue (some minor singing on the bottoms of their feet), however, their insusceptible framework doesn't react with a consume (rankling, torment, and so forth.) because their brains advise their bodies how to respond.

This is the way to progress. Your body does your convictions. Your convictions direct your activities, which thusly shape your experience. Some depict this procedure as making your prosperity or making your involvement with life. In our way of life, we see this portrayed inside the persuasive and positive mental demeanor writing. It very well may be seen in numerous regions of power. You can likewise think back to the people of yore and see it depicted in the particulars of the verifiable period. An individual a lot more astute than we are stated, "It will be done unto you as indicated by your conviction." In the current period of integrative medication and brain research, we call it self-hypnosis or mind-body medication. There are currently various logical examinations that show stunning outcomes for torment control, wound mending, physical change, and a lot more medical advantages than we recently suspected conceivable.

You can pick your beliefs. You may decide to accept what you see, in the feeling of "See it to trust it" or "Truth can be stranger than fiction." This is truly simple to do. You experience something with your faculties, and that is a natural method of picking whether it is reasonable or not. In any case, you may likewise decide to trust it first and afterward observe it, which may require some training. A great many people think that its simpler to let the world mention to them what is valid or what to accept.

The TV, media, papers, books, educators, and specialists besiege us with what to accept. You grew up finding out about the world and yourself from numerous outside sources. This prompted a recognizable example of watching and getting data about the world from outside yourself, and you picked which data to make a piece of your conviction framework. This included convictions about your body. For instance, when your stomach makes a thundering sound, you accept that it implies you are eager. Or on the other hand, you feel queasy and trust you are wiped out. Both of these are instances of watched occasions: you watched an association once and decided to trust it. In The Self-Hypnosis Diet, we are recommending that you turn that training around with this thought: "Trust it and you will see it." This implies you initially pick what to accept, and afterward, your body follows up on it as obvious and makes it genuine as far as you can tell.

One of the significant messages we trust you will get from this book is that your brain-body hears all that you hear, all that you state, all that you think, picture, or envision in your psyche, and it can't differentiate between what is genuine and what you envision. It follows up on what you need, accepts it, and anticipate. In light of this, which of these announcements would assist you with encountering the ideal weight you want: "I simply take a gander at food and put on weight" or "I can eat anything and my weight remains the equivalent"? Without a doubt the last mentioned. Be that as it may, which articulation do you accept to be valid for you?

Once more, it will be done unto you as per your conviction. We will assist you with the thoughts, language, and pictures that define successful sleep-inducing recommendations, however, you have complete authority over what you decide to accept. As you read the thoughts in this book and hear the sleep-inducing recommendations offered during the trancework on the sound, you will settle on numerous decisions for yourself. We wholeheartedly urge you to decide to trust it so you will see it for yourself. Your mind (mind-body) can't differentiate and will follow up on what you select in any case. Why not select what you truly need?

Emotions and Affirmations

Not all contemplations and convictions show themselves into your experience. Just those that have the vitality of your sentiments (feelings), alongside your conviction and your desire that something will occur, will show themselves. Your sentiments or feelings are a type of vitality that impacts this procedure of creation. That is, the point at which you have a solid inclination about a conviction, it contains vitality. That vitality makes your experience and further strengthens your convictions and desires. We are discussing the consolidated vitality of your considerations, your convictions, your desires, and what you need. The psychological vitality behind what you need and the amount you let yourself need it makes inspiration. So maybe you can see that it is critical to let yourself genuinely need something with extraordinary inclination. If you join feeling with need, you engage the procedure you are setting into movement inside you.

Ensure that your emotions stay positive. You can decide when they are certain or negative by how they affect you. It's basic. Feelings that cause you to feel great are certain, and feelings that cause you to feel awful are negative. Keep these energies positive by liking your needing (want), convictions, and desires. If you have negative musings and feelings, they will harm your inspiration. On the off chance that you have positive contemplations and feelings, they will fortify your inspiration.

Contemplations, convictions, and desires are equivalent to open door energies. You can draw in them and produce positive or negative impacts and results. If you are negative, anticipate negative outcomes. If you are certain, anticipate positive outcomes. As such any idea, conviction, or desire creates a negative or positive outcome. It's an easy decision—if you need achievement, look for positive vitality from positive contemplations and sentiments

Choosing Affirmations for Weight loss
Your mind-body likewise see your conviction dependent on your hidden inclination. Here is a model. Let us state that you need to think about something that will assist you with accomplishing your objective. You make a certification and start saying it out loud to yourself. Attestations are an awesome method to make positive thoughts and convictions. Talking assertions permits your ears to hear your voice talk them. This also is a method of picking your convictions and fortifying them. For instance, you may state the certification, "I am lighter and more slender today." But what do you feel? On the off chance that you "believe" you are overweight or feel that the attestation is false, and disclose to yourself the assertion, in any case, there is a contention. What you feel is another way that your inner mind sees your conviction or what you hold as obvious. Significantly, your sentiments are in arrangement with your confirmations and your wants, convictions, and desires. Keep in mind, feelings (emotions) are vitality. You might be asking, "However consider the possibility that I don't accept what I am letting myself know?" Do

it at any rate. It is superior to centering the vitality of your feelings, wants, and convictions in a negative way. It is additionally a stage toward the path you need to continue.

Self-Love for Weight Loss

Forgiveness is a significant improvement in cherishing yourself. At whatever point your excuse, you are "giving forward" or "giving up" of something you were holding inside you. Let us get straight to the point about this: pardoning is just for you, not any other person. It's anything but a type of tolerating, excusing or defending another person's activities. It is a procedure of relinquishing a negative inclination that has remained inside you dreadfully long. It is relinquishing any feeling or felt that may be an obstruction among you and cherishing yourself and having what you need. A large number of us are significantly more basic and a lot harder on ourselves than we are on others. At the point when you clutch contemplations of what you ought to or ought not to have done, you are not cherishing yourself. Rather, you are placing cognizant vitality into negative convictions about yourself. Contemplations, for example, "I ought to have gone for a stroll yesterday" or "I shouldn't have eaten that second bit of pie" may likewise be viewed as self-punishing. Sometimes, rebuffing yourself, either through the absence of eating or gorging, can even bring about dismissal for your wellbeing.

By moving your regard for self-thankfulness, you move from the negative to the positive, which is significantly more helpful for self-cherishing. Writing in a diary about the sound decisions you make every day can advance self-love. By pardoning yourself and excusing others, you discharge the enthusiastic hold that past occasions may have had on you, and you make yourself accessible to adore yourself. At the point when you discharge the impacts of past encounters by pardoning, you at that point experience genuine feelings of serenity and a quiet unwinding in your body that assist you with tolerating your ideal weight.

How to start loving your body
One reason we talk such a great amount about adoring yourself is because that is the place your self-acknowledgment needs to start. If you don't cherish yourself presently, in any event, having the attractive looks of a Paul Newman or a Marilyn Monroe can't offer that to you. Incidentally, did you realize that Marilyn Monroe wore a size 14? Remain before a mirror and take a gander at your body. Start with your head and work down through each piece of your body.

1. Review a portion of the things this body part has accomplished for you.

2. Tell it "thank you" for something explicit that it accomplished for you.

3. Proceed to the following body part.

4. In the wake of arriving at your feet and toes, return to your head.

Continue down your body, telling each body part, "I love you." You are in transit.

Since these cases are from our mind-body medication practice, let us quickly take a gander at a portion of the average ways that states of being are produced by the mind-body. There are numerous models wherein smothered and quelled feelings discover articulation by showing physical indications and conditions. Feelings and passionate clashes that are not intentionally recognized, communicated, or given voice can or will be communicated by the physical body. Here is a typical model.

At the point when outrage isn't recognized and communicated, it might cause muscles in the head, neck, and shoulders to fix and tense, which thus makes a pressure migraine. This is the exact articulation of a person or thing that is a genuine annoyance. Someone else encountering similar sentiments of outrage may be wrecking over the circumstance, and experience acid reflux, heartburn, or a fever. The skin is an organ that is exceptionally receptive to feelings, and a state of urticaria (hives) may emit when somebody is getting under their skin or annoying them or when the individual is tingling to do or say something, or some feeling is emitting to the surface.

Your feelings are your emotions, for example, glad, dismal, or irate. At the point when feelings or sentiments are not communicated, the brain-body will reflect them in inventive manners. Remedially, representations assist us with disentangling and comprehend what the body is communicating.

A saying or analogy portraying an enthusiastic response, for example, "a genuine annoyance" is communicated through muscle strain and cerebral pain because the passionate dissatisfaction isn't being communicated something else. This is a continuous encounter since commonly it isn't worthy or prudent to recognize and communicate outrage or different sentiments. For instance, if your chief humiliates you or makes an irrational solicitation, you could endanger your business if you communicated your displeasure. Rather, you put it out of mind and go on to something different. Putting it out of the brain doesn't put it out of the body. As you will find in the instances of hypnosis utilized in treatment, feelings and enthusiastic clashes can be put out of the brain, however not really out of the body.

I might want to depict the distinction among sentiments and considerations. Contemplations are thoughts, convictions, and decisions in your cognizant or "thinking mind." Feelings or feelings are communicated genuinely in your body. They begin from a crude territory somewhere down in the cerebrum called the limbic framework. The two contemplations and feelings are "things" as they are not simply in your brain. They include vitality and science, and they are transmitted genuinely and vigorously through your sensory system and different pathways in your body. The compound substances called synapses, for example, serotonin, dopamine, noradrenaline, and acetylcholine, are the more typical ones included.

Find comfort in yourself

Let us take a gander at another case that represents another basic passionate subject that happened by the brain-body in weight issues. Mary depicted a lifetime of picking up and losing what she called "a similar twenty-five pounds of weight." When we took her history, she said that her weight issues started when she set off for college and repeated with each geographic move and with every relationship change. At age thirty-six, Mary was accomplished and settled on astute decisions about her food and eating conduct. She was effective in all aspects of her life and was puzzled regarding why she was unable to be fruitful in shedding pounds. She had perused a few books about hypnosis and needed to utilize it to reveal to her body to lose the weight. Mary went into a casual condition of daze without any problem. We offered trancelike recommendations to assist her with finding if there were any obstructions or boundaries to her weight reduction.

That is, we inquired as to whether there was a purpose behind recovering and keeping the weight that she wished to lose. Pictures of fourth grade struck a chord. Mary portrayed a warm spring day when she was nine years of age, strolling home from grade school. Showing up home, she pulled out the key her mom gave her that morning so she could give herself access to the house. Mary's mom had relinquished her position as a medical attendant when Mary was conceived. This was the principal day of her mom's arrival to her nursing profession, and this was the first run through Mary had returned home to an unfilled house.

In my office, Mary started to cry as she felt so forlorn without her mother there to welcome her in the kitchen, although she realized her mother would be home in under 60 minutes. She strolled through the house, feeling a blend of deadness and forlornness. She depicted the physical impression of being "unfilled" in her stomach. Back in the kitchen, she found a note on the kitchen table with her name on it. It stated, "Hello, Honey, I will be home soon. I put some pudding in the cooler for you. Love, Mommy." Mary was presently half chuckling, half crying as she disclosed to me that she could even taste the solace of that vanilla pudding at this moment, here in the workplace. Afterward, she worked out an order of her weight and the relationship to geographic moves, work changes, and relationship changes. She saw her example of eating desserts, (for example, pudding and different treats) during the occasions she expected to fill the vacancy when forlorn or while missing what or whom she left at whatever point she moved. Mary found what she expected to change, so food didn't need to fill the passionate vacancy any longer.

I might want to introduce the possibility of an enthusiastic continuum, where one end is negative feelings and the furthest edge is sure feelings. On the negative end are the sentiments of blame, disgrace, disdain, outrage, despise, and dread. At the positive finish of the continuum are joy, happiness, delight, sympathy, satisfaction, harmony, and love. As with the impacts of feelings, we might want you to consider them either positive or negative, with the negative end called dread, and the positive end called love. Lessen every one of the feelings to its delegate impact of advancing either dread or love.

At the point when you distinguish the individual feelings and their belongings as dread or love—either—it will be simpler for you to pick the ones you need and to discharge the ones you don't need. Eating for enthusiastic reasons has, at its center, the endeavor to dispose of dread. By picking the positive, you produce the good conditions for bliss, which supports your ideal weight. Partner your eating with the positive feelings (love) is one method of unlearning the negative examples of eating and regarding food as adoration. It is fine to adore your food, yet don't make food a substitute for affection and the other positive feelings. Challenge and delete the negative feelings (dread) with what they require, which isn't food.

Chapter 6:

Guided Meditations for Weight Loss

The way to your ideal weight will presumably be full of traps, land mines, and saboteurs. Any commendable objective has deterrents to be survived. This section is tied in with perceiving those obstructions, excusing some of them, and making an intense move to dispense with the others. The entrancing trancework centers around contemplations and thoughts at the brain-body level that will empower the procedure. Acquaint yourself with contemplations, old examples of conduct, extraordinary get-togethers, and regular settings that may attack your ideal weight. This is the initial move toward making the way to your ideal weight. When you can perceive the triggers to indulging, you just need to rehearse approaches to handily excuse those inconvenient hindrances. On the off chance that this appears to be overpowering, don't stress. As we've stated, we will direct you in your trancework, so you may convey precisely what you need to state to your glorious psyche body.

Understand where you are right now
As you start your way, evaluate where you are present. New numbers from the United States Government's National Health and Nutrition Examination Survey (NHANES) affirm that overweight and corpulence are

as yet a significant general wellbeing concern. As indicated by information from 1999 to 2002, 65.1 percent of grown-ups matured twenty or more established were overweight or corpulent. The pace of stoutness was 30.4 percent, and 4.9 percent of U.S. grown-ups were incredibly stout. Overweight is characterized as having a weight record (BMI) of 25 or higher. Heftiness is having a BMI of 30 or higher. Having a BMI of 40 or higher is extraordinary corpulence.

To decide your BMI: Divide your weight (in pounds) by the square of your tallness (in inches) and afterward duplicate that number by 703. Remember that an individual who is solid with a low muscle to fat ratio may have a higher BMI since muscle gauges more than fat. In this way, on the off chance that you are 5'8" and weigh 185 pounds, your BMI is 28. To see where you are at present, contrasted and different Americans, take a gander at these insights: Nearly 66% of U.S. grown-ups are overweight (BMI of 25 or higher, which incorporates the large individuals). Almost 33% of U.S. grown-ups are fat (BMI of 30 or higher). Not exactly 50% of U.S. grown-ups have a solid weight (BMI higher than or equivalent to 18.5 and lower than 25).

Shielding your prosperity and making the way start with you. As you read in the prior sections, everything starts with contemplations and convictions about what you need, how you need it, and what you can accept and acknowledge. All self-crushing musings must be killed and changed into insistences of your prosperity. For instance, on the off chance that you persistently state, "My stomach is the greatest piece of my concern," what are you telling your psyche body? What is your psyche body going to make valid for you? Here is the attestation that kills and changes that announcement and different articulations like it: "My body is entirely formed." When you experience contemplations that don't bolster your ideal weight, recollect this certification, and follow these four stages.

1. You should trust it is feasible for you to have the ideal weight you want.

2. You should need it and feel you merit it.

3. Acknowledge any demand as a chance to have your ideal weight.

4. Let yourself expect the outcomes you want, and invest in expelling any snag from inside or without.

Let go of old patterns
Examples of conduct with food, eating, and exercise must turn out to be progressively good with the outcomes you need. Here are a few different ways to begin moving your point of view:

• If you love low-quality nourishment, you should relinquish an everyday diet of shoddy nourishment and welcome some new, more advantageous food sources that help your solid weight.

• If you have an antipathy for practice and physical movement, you should invite the every day physical action that excites and fortifies your body.

The equivalent is valid for the subliminally determined examples that make desires. You start by distinguishing contradictory longings as obstructions and imprint them for evacuation. This tells your subliminal that it has your authorization to follow up for your benefit. The trancework contains recommendations that enable you to invite new examples of conduct.

There is no reason that legitimizes an obstruction to your prosperity. This incorporates any reason about the costs related with weight reduction. Truly, quality nourishments may cost more than inexpensive food, however your ideal weight merits each penny and each pound lighter. We have had patients reveal to us that get-healthy plans are excessively costly or that their medical coverage won't spread the costs of a get-healthy plan. No measure of cash is a substantial reason to shield you from making progress. The ailments related with overabundance weight will cost you more over the long haul. On the off chance that your interest in the issue exceeds your interest in the arrangement, you will keep the issue.

Fixations on food or weight can be obstructions to fruitful sound weight. To break these examples, make strong move to defuse, kill, or change any fanatical considerations, for example, "I'm generally ravenous," "All I consider is food," or "I need to eat." This may mean conversing with an instructor in the event that it is a fixation that warrants clinical intercession. On the off chance that you feel that you can't change over the top contemplations without anyone else, you will most likely profit by proficient assistance.

Try not to rationalize in light of the fact that you believe you need self discipline. On the off chance that you have the self discipline to inhale clean air or read this book, you have the determination fundamental for everything else you need in your life. Become touchy to the reasons you hear others utilizing, the reasons that they state they can't have what they need. Give specific consideration to people who are overweight as they talk about the deterrents to their weight reduction.

Mind and Metabolic Problems
Another regular metabolic impediment is the weight-gain impacts related with stimulant drug treatment. Antidepressants come in three significant classes: tricyclics (e.g., amitriptyline, for example, Elavil), particular serotonin reuptake inhibitors (SSRIs, for

example, Paxil and Zoloft), and monoamine oxidase inhibitors (MAOIs, considerably less now and again utilized). Each can influence hunger, starch longings, and metabolic changes that expand weight. On the off chance that you are utilizing an upper, you might need to converse with your doctor about utilizing the most minimal viable measurement, since it is typically the higher doses that cause the best issue with weight gain. Opiates are another class of medications that can impact weight gain. Opiate analgesics (torment relievers) have two factors that may influence weight.

Initially, all sedative subsidiaries or opiates depressingly affect the focal sensory system, which causes the common peristalsis, or wavelike movement through the stomach related framework, to back off, which thus may slow different parts of digestion. Second, people with torment typically have versatility issues that limit their physical movement. For a few, the CNS (focal sensory system) depressant impacts may restrain physical movement much further. A portion of the nonnarcotic meds may have options, yet likewise with stimulant utilize noted before, the successful portion and medication is the main goal.

Any individual who has encountered a physical issue that limits physical movement realizes how rapidly weight can increment. People with incapacities or impediments that restrict or block physical movement and exercise must be innovative in such a manner. A devouring mental test can once in a while influence weight reduction. Although we have no experimental research to prove the connection between exhausting mental vitality and weight reduction, we do think it merits considering. For instance, taking a class that requires extreme mental vitality may expend calories and fill in as an option in contrast to eating improperly. Another thought may be to talk with a physical or word related advisor and investigate innovative approaches to fortify those pieces of the body than can be effectively moved.

Procrastination

Procrastination is the purposeful and ongoing delay of doing things that you state you need to do. It is certainly a type of self-harm. Tarrying is the decision to not do what will move you to your objective of flawless weight. There are numerous systems for managing to dawdle. If you are hesitating about transforming from an inactive to a functioning way of life, start by strolling around the area for fifteen minutes consistently, instead of focusing on an overwhelming 60 minutes, five-times-each week wellness focus plan. Start little, and take on additional as you feel great and prepared. Do it such that suits you. Maybe you have a character that would prefer to focus on making a plunge without removing time to think yourself from it. Or on the other hand, it may be useful to discover an accomplice who will invigorate you to do it until you unlearn the old conduct. I like the Nike trademark: "Take care of business."

Keep in mind, your weight isn't the aftereffect of the mix-ups you have made; it is just the undesirable consequence of how you have been living. An ongoing Yankelovich Preventative Healthcare Study reviewed 6,000 grown-up Americans with respect to issues of wellbeing. It found that near 65 percent of Americans have never gone to a sustenance class, and 50 percent have never taken a wellness class. Since 65 percent of Americans are overweight, could there be a connection between's being overweight and the nonattendance of data about sustenance and wellness? We suspect as much.

Presently how about we take a gander at the hindrances in your way that others present. These deterrents remember the conspicuous and concealed saboteurs for your everyday existence with loved ones, at office get-togethers, at uncommon get-togethers and occasions, while voyaging and eating out, while being an objective for weight separation, and in your kitchen. These snags essentially include others, yet at the same time require some activity and consideration on your part to secure your ideal weight. You simply need to turn out to be increasingly acquainted with the opportunities for harm and practice how to best deal with any person or thing that "assaults you from behind." fortunately you, at last, are answerable for your decisions in every one of these circumstances. The daze takes a shot at the sound will offer recommendations that advise your inner mind-body approaches to deal with conceivable damage.

With our customers, we have seen that regularly the best type of treachery will be originated from those nearest to you, your loved ones. On the off chance that you have been on a careful nutritional plan previously, you think about eating routine saboteurs. Maybe they have good intentions, maybe not. Change isn't simple for everybody, and when you declare that you have made changes to your eating schedule, others may not comprehend what that implies for them or what changes this may force upon them. They will swear by the comfortable schedules with you that they have known before.

At the point when others appear to undermine your endeavors, you should decide why they are carrying on in opposition to your objectives. If it is the change, at that point maybe they mean well however simply don't yet comprehend what to do to help you. A couple of expressive words that clarify benevolently and unmistakably your new aims will do ponders here. "I realize I used to consistently have a twofold scoop of strawberry frozen yogurt after supper, however now I possibly eat when I'm eager ... thus, perhaps later I'll have a scoop." Or "Really, I brought over an incredible new treat: strawberry sorbet."

How meditation can help burn fat

Where do you store most of your fat? Your paunch? Provided that this is true, we have news for you. While the vast majority of our muscle versus fat (subcutaneous) is the wiggly, jiggly kind that we can see and squeeze — there exists an inconspicuous, more profound, increasingly vile sort of fat which goes past essentially making our preferred sweater a piece excessively cozy.

What sort of damage would it be able to do? So ruinous, this stuff adheres to our organs, wrenches up our pressure hormones, sets our body burning with irritation — while additionally being connected to hypertension, diabetes, coronary illness, certain malignant growths, and even cerebrum issue like dementia.

"Be that as it may, I'm generally slim, this stuff doesn't influence me, correct? I don't have anything to stress over."

Reconsider. One investigation found that slim individuals who ate right yet didn't practice had heaps of instinctive fat. On the off chance that you have surrender to an existence of being "thin fat" at that point you may be in danger.

Have you attempted each midsection fat dissolving diet and exercise routine without much of any result? Would you be able to lose fat wherever on your body aside from your difficult waist? All things considered, it probably won't be your flaw. As per specialists at the University of Massachusetts (Hardy et al), with worry as a main source, a high level of individuals with abundance midsection fat can accuse their situation for what's known as "insulin obstruction."

I'm not catching this' meaning, precisely?

At the point when our insulin receptors don't open up appropriately, our liver and muscle cells can't store the vitality (glucose) we need from food. This sends our glucose to the moon.

The entirety of this additional vitality's gotta' head off to some place. Also, it does... it gets changed over to fat. In any case, not the ordinary delicate and cushioned kind that really reacts well to abstain from food and exercise.

The expanse of glucose flowing in insulin safe individuals' circulation system turns into the famously undesirable previously mentioned instinctive fat. Adhering like insane paste to our midriff and essential organs, the best answer for instinctive fat might just be a stick of explosive. Intensifying the issue, with starving, healthfully insufficient cells — insulin safe individuals regularly have an unquenchable craving.

Since their blood markers are not exactly in the pre-diabates/diabetes run, these people regularly hang in clinical limbo, undiscovered by their primary care physician. While the proven techniques for focusing on ultra-difficult stomach fat are a low-sugar diet (Paleo, Mediterranean, and so on) and specific sorts of activity (High Intensity Interval Training HIIT), there exists an under the radar dull pony.

While contemplation is the exact opposite thing a great many people consider with regards to consuming stomach fat, the investigations demonstrate something else.

In what capacity can a training that to a great extent focuses on the mind be so compelling at burning obstinate tummy fat? Since meditation captures the mystery detestable operator liable for insulin opposition: stress.

Incredibly, the investigation found that the individuals who were exceptionally mindful of their musings and sentiments (as estimated by MAAS) really gauged considerably less in general (BMI), and all the more incredibly, when put under a powerful x-beam scanner — likewise had signficantly less stomach fat than the benchmark group!

Turning into a driving force repairman through meditation does substantially more than essentially make you quiet, brilliant, and centered — it can truly overhaul your body.

3 Ways You Can Make Learning to Meditate Easier

Hopping into contemplation can be scary. What precisely would you say you should do while you stay there? It is safe to say that you should think or not think? Would it be advisable for you to check your breaths? To what extent would it be a good idea for you to contemplate? Here are three hints that will make figuring out how to ruminate simpler.

1. Pick a Meditation App

Guided meditation is the most ideal path for a tenderfoot to begin pondering. In guided contemplation, you're ordinarily given guidelines and a concentration for the meeting. There hushes up an ideal opportunity for you to work on reflecting, yet the guide occasionally checks in and afterward wraps up the meeting.

2. Timetable Your Meditation

This is the part I battle with the most. A characteristic time for reflecting is before anything else. It establishes a brilliant pace for the afternoon. You are less inclined to put off pondering on the off chance that you make a propensity for doing it toward the beginning of the day. Be that as it may, morning contemplation doesn't work for me since everybody in my family is up right on time, and I don't have an uncommon intercession space in the house where no one will trouble me. During the school year, I have the house to myself from 8:00 am to 2:30 pm, with the goal that's the point at which I attempt to fit in contemplation. At the point when that is outlandish, I in some cases reflect after the children head to sleep. All things considered, the meditation is all the more a slowing down exercise, instead of an equipping.

It's simple for your contemplation practice to tumble to the base of the rundown since it appears to be so inefficient. Notwithstanding, the greater part of us — myself included—effectively squander at any rate ten minutes via web-based networking media consistently. During this combative political race season, web-based life can be a noteworthy wellspring of stress. As opposed to tumbling down a bunny gap of governmental issues, settle on a choice to step away and center around the current second.

3. Set Your Intention

The advantages of contemplation can regularly be difficult to evaluate or even depict. On the off chance that you lift loads, you can see your muscles develop, however it is extremely unlikely for us to see our amplified tactile cortex. The impact of expanded care on your weight won't be quick or emotional, so this methodology requires persistence and a capacity to take the long view. Hence, you may wind up getting baffled if you begin pondering to get in shape.

Rather than having an objective for meditation, concoct an aim. Aims are increasingly about the current second, not about some future achievement or disappointment. One may be, "associate with friends and family," or "remain quiet," or "discover harmony." You will probably discover different advantages of meditation, yet attempt to remain concentrated on the day by day practice, not the final product.

Figure out how to Listen to Yourself
Meditation is anything but an enchantment weight reduction arrangement. You should have great sustenance propensities, fuse development in your life, and get satisfactory rest. Nonetheless, figuring out how to contemplate can assist you with figuring out how to focus on your body's signs of yearning and satiety, which will manage your eating and assist you with getting a charge out of the food you devour.

Chapter 7:

100 Positive Affirmations to lose weight

1. My self-esteem increase by losing weight
Confidence comes from within. There are certain that increases confidence and self-esteem. My self-esteem and confidence increase from losing the extra calories my body owns. As I lose the extra body fat, my confidence boosts. My self-esteem reaches to a high level as my weight drops.

2. I achieve my weight loss goals every day
Whenever I plan to pull anything off, I tend to set small goals in order to achieve a bigger one. The weight loss journey is a long journey and setting small goals help to achieve it. I set small goals every day like do 50 push-ups and next day 100, achieving these small goals every day motivates me throughout the journey and helps me to achieve my bigger goal.

3. I like to exercise daily
Exercise is the best way to reduce weight. I love to exercise. It makes me healthy and helps to burn the extra calories. Exercise increases my metabolism that eventually cuts off the extra calories. Exercise not only reduces my weight, but it also lowers the chances of diseases such as cancer. It also prevents heart attack.

4. I love to eat healthy food

Vegetables and Fruits are very beneficial to our health. They are low in fat and high in fibres. Fibres help to digest food. I personally like to eat that are helpful to my wellbeing and health. I prefer eating eggs and fish. I avoid red meat and oil food that are not good for health.

5. I avoid snacks and fast food

I do not prefer eating snacks or fast food. I only eat when I am hungry. Fast food and snacks consist of unhealthy fats that increase body calories. I tend to avoid it. I choose healthy food over delicious food. It greatly helps to maintain my weight.

6. I have finally achieved my ideal weight

Whenever I achieve small goals and then eventually the bigger one that is weight loss. I appreciate myself and constantly keeps myself in a positive state of mind. I remind myself that my hard work really paid off and I achieved my goal.

7. I love binging to healthy food

Healthy food has numerous benefits. From weight loss to glowing skin, healthy food provides you with every benefit. Healthy food consists of multiple items that are fruits, vegetables, pulses, grains, and fish as well. All of the things mentioned taste marvellous and are extremely good for health. They greatly help in losing weight.

8. I control my diet

I now clearly know when to eat and when to not. I know that when my body wants liquids and when something solid. Most of the times, we are not actually hungry but we confuse our thirst and need for water with something solid. I control myself and only eat when I am actually hungry.

9. I enjoy doing workout a lot

Work out and exercise make me feel very good. It increases my metabolism and cuts off the excessive calories. I burn my extra calories off with the help of work out. Work out makes me active and fast. My muscles become strong with the help of work out.

10. My body is becoming stronger every day through exercise

Exercise and work out has a very positive effect on my body. It has made my body stronger and fitter than before. I feel much fresh and active after the workout. The work out helps to sweat out the extra fat.

11. I am maintaining my ideal weight

With the help of a balanced diet and everyday work out, I am able to maintain my ideal weight. Losing weight is easy but maintaining it requires hard work. I maintain my ideal weight by consuming a healthy diet. Exercise and work out keep my weight at an ideal level.

12. I love my body

I am the person who should love myself the most. If I will love myself then others will too. I love being myself. I love to maintain myself and take care of myself. I care for my body because health is wealth.

13. I am worthy of a healthy, good-looking and slim body

My body should look appealing to others. It should be healthy and smart. I deserve to look attractive and smart. I feel confident when I look attractive and smart. My social life boosts when I look attractive.

14. I prefer eating healthy than junk

Junk food is great for the taste buds but they are not good for the stomach and health. They tend to make the immune system weak. When the body's immune system is weak, it is more vulnerable to diseases. I prefer healthy food over junk to avoid such fuss.

15. I lose weight every day

When I choose healthy food over the junk food and do work out regularly then extra fat of my body burns every day. When I lose extra fat every day then I get slimmer every day. This thought makes very excited and pushes me to maintain my weight.

16. I feel great when I look great

Our appearances matter a lot. It matters to the outside world and it matters to us as well. When you look great, everyone compliments you and consequently, you feel great. Looking great and feeling great has a deep connection.

17. I love being healthy and attractive

I try to do whatever it takes to look attractive. The key to looking attractive is to be healthy. When you are healthy, you are automatically attractive. From drinking healthy juices to doing yoga in the morning, I do everything to maintain my health and weight.

18.   I redefined success

Success is not having 6 digit amount of money in your bank account. The money cannot give you happiness if you are not healthy. I have redefined success by achieving my ideal weight. Not only achieving it but also maintaining it.

19. I meditate every day

Doing yoga and meditation helps to keep toxins out of the body. I meditate every day to keep my body healthy and good-looking. I choose healthy lifestyle techniques to look and feel attractive.

20.   I consume foods that are beneficial for me

Food has a very important impact on your life. Your body and skin show what you eat. Whatever you consume, appears on your skin. Due to this, I try to intake foods that are healthy and beneficial for my body. When my body feels good consequently I feel good. I prefer taking food that is low in fat and good for my health.

21.My health depends on me

I have always been a person who loves to take extra care of everything. I am not a careless person regarding my health and body. I clearly understand that I am responsible for my health. This means that I should take steps that are beneficial to my health.

22.   I embrace my body

I constantly appreciate myself for the efforts I do for maintaining my health and body. As I lose weight and reaches to the ideal body weight, I love my body more. I embrace it every moment.

23.   I choose to stay patient during the weight loss journey

Patience is the key to achieve big goals. Every work requires patience. Patience and persistence make the person accomplish the goals. I try to remain patient during the journey. Patience makes it easier for me to achieve my goal.

24.   I enjoy early morning workouts a lot

I look forward to early morning workouts every day. They make my skin and body fresh. Work out not only makes my skin fresh it also helps me to lose weight. Work out makes my body to lose extra fat. When my body loses extra fat then it becomes fitter and better.

25. I am strictly following my weight loss plan

Whenever you need to achieve something, the first step is to create a plan. A proper plan leads to the completion of the task. The most important plan of my life right now is weight loss. This plan mainly depends on switching my eating habits from unhealthy to healthy.

26. I appreciate my efforts during the weight loss journey

Controlling oneself is a hard task. Controlling your appetite and cravings while losing weight is a difficult job. This is more difficult when you are a person who loves food. But if you want to lose weight and look attractive then you have to overcome your eating habit. I have successfully done this and I am proud of myself on having control on myself.

27. I am healthier and slimmer than the previous day

During the weight loss journey, I have adopted such habits that not only helped me to lose weight but also made me healthier. The habits such as doing yoga, meditation, exercise, eating healthy food, and avoiding junk. They have greatly helped me to lose weight. You can also adopt such habits and welcome a healthy life.

28. I am ready to welcome my attractive body

The key to an attractive body is to eliminate unhealthy patterns from your life. The unhealthy patterns of life are intaking food that is high in sugar, high in fats, and not doing exercise. I have eliminated such patterns from my life and now I am readily towards the path to get an attractive body.

29.   I say no to junk food

Junk food is the culprit of most of the diseases. Junk food leads to obesity that is one of the major problems of the world. I try my best to avoid junk food. If you want to lose weight and want a good-looking body then you should also steer clear of junk food.

30.   I prefer eating fresh fruits in order to get a healthy body

Fresh fruits have minerals and fibres that are extremely healthy for the body. They are high in nutrients and low in calories. They help to increase immunity. Fruits have antioxidants that boost health. I have developed a habit of eating fresh fruits because I want a healthy and sound body.

31. I have adopted a healthy lifestyle

Your lifestyle has a very big impact on your health. Bad and careless lifestyle such as disturbed sleep cycle, consuming junk food, and not doing exercise leads to an unhealthy body. On the other hand, getting appropriate sleep, doing exercise, and eating healthy food gives you a healthy body. I have successfully adopted a healthy lifestyle.

32.   I am enjoying my healthy lifestyle

My healthy lifestyle is assuring me a healthy and fit body. I am getting a glow and achieving my ideal weight with the help of my healthy lifestyle. While following my healthy lifestyle, I feel good because the outcome is according to my wish.

33.   I have achieved an ideal body due to a healthy lifestyle

Healthy lifestyle such as doing exercise daily and intaking healthy food leads to the ideal body. I have able to get ideal body because of my healthy lifestyle. I am strictly following my healthy lifestyle and have welcomed my ideal body.

34.   I adore my ideal body

I love and adore my ideal body. I have lost the extra fat of my body and now I fit into my favourite clothes easily. I love to check out myself in the mirror every day. I appreciate my efforts each day.

35.   I enjoy being in my ideal body

Nothing makes me happier than the fact that I have accomplished my goal of losing weight. By losing some of the extra fats of my body, I have achieved an ideal body. I feel marvellous when people compliment me.

36.   My eating habits are improving my body

I have adopted healthy eating habits that have transformed my body. Eating healthy is the key to a healthy life and healthy life means a healthy body. Eating healthy is defined as to add a lot of vegetables and fruits to your menu.

37. I have lost extra pounds of my body to impress my girlfriend

I have always been a person who is conscious about the looks and personality. The extra pounds on the body use to make me complexed in front of people. I have successfully lost extra pounds to make my girl happy.

38. I cannot wait to meet my girlfriend with my ideal body

I have achieved my long-awaited goal that was weight loss. Now I am very excited to meet my girlfriend and show her my new ideal body. She will be so proud of me as I am proud of myself.

39. I have achieved a flat stomach

Due to regular exercise and consuming healthy food I have been able to get a flat stomach. I have achieved a flat stomach and now I am more confident. My self-esteem has boosted.

40. I have successfully reduced my appetite

I only eat when I am hungry. I have cut off the snacks from my life. I try to eat food that is low in fat and full of minerals. I have trained my stomach to eat less.

41.I am proudly weighing 15 pounds less
When I use the weighing machine, it made me proud that I have lost many pounds. These pounds were like an extra burden on my body. After losing the extra pounds of my body, I feel more confident than ever.

42.	I look forward to taking a walk in the park every day
Jogging and morning walk makes me active and fresh. I have made a routine to do jogging in the morning. By doing this I inhale the fresh air in the morning. It makes my skin glow and burns off the extra fat of my body.

43.	I love doing toning exercise minimum 4 times a week
I love doing exercise a lot. Toning exercise makes my body lean and strong. I try to do toning exercise as much as I can. It is a must in my daily routine. Sometimes if the office work makes me tired then I miss it but I try to do it a minimum 4 times during the week.

44.	I stay hydrated
Water makes the body fresh and glowing. I help to remove the toxins out of the body. The excretory system is also regulated by the water.

45.	I love to drink plenty of water
Water is very essential in the weight loss journey. It tends to suppress the appetite if taken before

the meal. Replace soda drinks with water and welcome the healthy body.

46.   I consume fresh vegetables and fruits daily

I have added fresh vegetables and fruits in my daily menu and it has improved my health a lot. Fruits and vegetables are very beneficial for health. They tend to make the body healthier and slimmer.

47.   I love to eat fish and chicken

Proteins are very important for health. In the weight loss journey, you have to cut off the carbohydrates and in order to compensate that you should take proteins. To fulfil my protein content, I count on chicken and fish.

48.   I count on emotional and mental skills for success

The emotional and mental state is very important in achieving any goal. I work on my emotional and mental state to keep me motivated during the journey. If your emotional and mental state is in a good state then it is easy for you to achieve your goal.

49.   I am using spiritual skills to accomplish my goal

Spiritual skills also play an important part in your daily life. Your spiritual skills should be good enough to keep you doing the great work. Spiritual skills are enhanced by doing yoga and other meditating techniques.

50. I am willing to change my body

Think and you have achieved your half goal. The moment you make up your mind, you have passed the half journey towards your goal. When I make up my mind to achieve something then I go every extreme to achieve it.

51. I am ready to create new thoughts about my body

Changing your body in a positive way is always a good chance. You should always brainstorm on the facts that how you can change your body. You should always be ready to create and construct new ways to transform your body.

52. I am willing to change my thinking about my myself

Welcome your new self every day. Every day you are achieving your weight loss goals. You should always be positive about yourself.

53. I appreciate my new self

As I have accomplished my goal of achieving ideal weight, I appreciate and adore myself more.

54. I love my new appearance

My new appearance is more attractive and alluring. I have an ideal weight and a flat stomach that makes me more confident.

55. I am very excited to try new and unique food

The journey of weight loss includes trying new food that I haven't tried before.

56. It is very exciting to try new food and exercise techniques for losing weight

Losing weight requires doing exercise and trying new food. This is very exciting and I enjoy this journey.

57. I am a motivation to others

I have lost some extra fat of my body by changing my lifestyle and others can take motivation from me.

58. I am a success story of weight loss

I have successfully lost weight in the past few days. My weight loss journey is a success story.

59. I enjoy following the healthy food plan

Healthy food plan includes consuming a lot of water, eating fruits and vegetables. The fresh fruits and vegetables taste marvellous and I enjoy eating them.

60. I love being at the ideal weight

My ideal weight makes me feel healthy and attractive.

61. I love making positive changes in my life

Eating healthy food and doing exercise are positive changes in my life. They have greatly helped me to lose weight.

62. I choose positive changes that help me to lose weight

I am proud of myself for making positive changes in my life. They contributed to my weight loss journey.

63.   I feel good while exercising

Exercise makes my body fresh and active. It makes my muscles strong.

64.   I enjoy music while exercising

I release my stress during exercise. Music helps me to release stress while exercising.

65.   I use relaxation techniques to handle the stress

Relaxation techniques such as deep breathing and yoga are great for handling the stress.

66.   I relax while doing deep breathing

Deep inhaling and exhaling help me to release stress. It makes my body healthy and stress-free.

67.   I am an attractive person with ideal body weight

My ideal body weight makes me attractive and good-looking person. After achieving my ideal body weight, I feel more attractive alluring

68.   I deserve to look charming and attractive

Losing weight is one of the great milestones of my life.

69.   I maintain myself at an ideal weight

I am strictly following a healthy lifestyle to maintain my ideal weight

70.   It is perfectly safe for me to lose some
        extra fat

Losing some fat off the body is healthy. Extra fat on the body increases cholesterol and leads to heart diseases. Losing fat off the body makes the body healthy.

71. I deserve everybody's love and care

When you look strong and fit then everybody loves you more.

72.   I am more fearless at my ideal weight

Ideal weight makes me more confident. My ideal weight increases my morale.

73.   I accept myself

I accept myself at my ideal weight. Every day I work hard to maintain it.

74.   I have improved my metabolism

By taking the fresh vegetables, my metabolism has improved a lot.

75.   I have a fast metabolism

With the help of a healthy diet, my metabolism has become fast.

76.   I try my best to maintain my weight at
        the ideal point

A healthy lifestyle has helped me to achieve an ideal weight. I make sure that I follow the healthy lifestyle strictly.

77. I know I can do this!

I keep myself motivated throughout the weight loss journey.

78. I count my body as my friend

As you know that health is the best wealth you can have. I try my best to maintain my healthy body.

79. I express myself through my appearance

My appearance says a lot about me. I make sure that I look charming and attractive.

80. I am willing to overcome the resistances

Every task requires hard work. I make sure to overcome every difficulty I face during the weight loss journey.

81. I am responsible for my present

seeing yourself as the saviour of your present will help you to analyse your mistakes and work for their betterment.

82. I am the originator of my future

We all tend to look at the bright side of what the future holds for us.

83. I believe in myself that I can lose weight

Belief and motivation go hand in hand. You need to believe in yourself that you will lose weight

84. I acknowledge my efforts in weight loss journey

giving yourself recognition in the weight loss journey is imperative. So, acknowledge your efforts and make progress each day

85.	I am approaching my ideal weight as each day passes

weight loss journey is a tiring one and you shed weight slowly. Seeing the progress and acknowledging it can be fruitful in the long run

86.	I enjoy being physically fit and strong

who does not want to have a fit and strong body? You need to have a positive mind-set and enjoy this journey of fat to fit.

87.	I lose weight every day to achieve my ideal weight

losing weight every day and seeing the progress will keep you motivated. Keep this positive thought in your mind so you can resist your favourite food.

88.	I know my metabolism helps me to achieve my ideal weight

have faith in your body to make progress and this is one of the best ways to stay motivated during your weight loss journey

89.	I have become a physically active person

You will start to feel more energized when you start your weight loss journey. Being physically active will also make your mind sharper.

90.	I properly chew the food so that it gets digested easily

Developing good eating habits will help you to keep your ideal weight for a longer time.

91.I do physical chores to achieve my ideal weight

staying active all day will keep you motivated and also help you complete many chores that you would ideally ignore

92.   I adore myself a lot

loving your body and soul is the key to losing weight and having a happy life.

93.   I appreciate being fit and active

give yourself some treat when you achieve a weight loss goal

94.   I have good control over my body weight

Staying off the bad carbs and encouraging good eating habits is important for losing weight.

95.   I feel attractive in my clothes

losing the extra pounds will make you confident about your body and you will start to look good in almost all the clothes.

96.   I say no to unhealthy food

keeping off the processed food and fast food will help you lose weight quickly.

97.   I binge eat food that is healthy for me

Veggies and food items with good nutritional value should be consumed more and you need to store this in your mind.

98.   I am proud of myself for achieving the weight loss goal

take pride in losing weight and you will feel like a winner. This confidence will then propel you in professional life.

99.   I am at peace knowing that I am at my ideal weight

losing weight will help you to keep the unwanted stress away and you will live a happy life.

100.   I feel my body shape is perfect and attractive

enjoy the body shape after losing some pounds. These small moments will motivate you further.

Chapter 8:

How to Practice Every Day Hypnosis

You cannot achieve your weight loss goal in a single day. I am still working on the program and have shed more than 20 pounds in three months. This is a constant struggle and you need to look at it as a part of your daily life. When you train your mind and body to achieve your desired weight, you will be able to regain your confidence and will see life with a new perspective. The affirmations and meditations are not only used for weight loss, they can overturn your negative mindset into a positive one. You will be able to achieve success in your personal and professional life as well. People tend to lose weight and then go back to their old eating habits, get lazy, and gain weight again. What I will explain in this chapter is how you can practice affirmations and meditations daily and also explain the process behind these daily routines.

Affirmations in mind
The more the desire contrasts from what your reality shows you, the more drawn out or more grounded the "affirmation" should be. When you have discovered a sentence, a recipe that deciphers your desire totally and genuinely, you can say this definition in your mind. Once or more than once. It's implied that it is smarter to rehash the desire. You can likewise while detailing your

desire in your mind, move your lips, which is progressively compelling. In some cases, it is simply impractical to state your desire for all to hear.

Saying the affirmations out loud
Saying the affirmations out loud is more impressive than in contemplations; in writing, we find that it is exceptionally powerful to state the confirmation out resoundingly before the mirror while looking at yourself without flinching. You can likewise do this in a soft tone, you can do it without pushing and it must be managed without the exertion of the will. In any case, I believe that when you say the affirmations out loud, it solidifies your belief on them. You will spend time and effort on this and this will strengthen your desire to lose weight and bring positivity in your life. You can likewise tune in to the plan on tape. At the point when you let it play around evening time, the affirmations go straightforwardly to the inner mind, which builds their viability.

Recording the affirmations
Recording the plan is the best way. It is the most impressive detailing to etch the idea in the inner mind. As said previously, believing is less incredible, saying your desire out loud is all the more impressive and recording it is the most remarkable way: it is a blend of visual and locomotory angles and it leaves something substantial. I developed a habit of saving the affirmations in a computer file and this process can also

help you keep a record of them. (Except if you sense that another content mirrors your requirements better, at that point you need to transform it and keep to these changes). You can compose the insistence on a card and take a look at it at whatever point you have the chance.

Representations for your daily life
There is another approach to make "affirmations" and that is to picture them. This implies you need to remember the picture of what you wish, as obviously as could reasonably be expected while envisioning yourself in the circumstance that you see, that you experience. This unavoidably implies envisioning the desire goes connected at the hip with feelings, with the delight one feels when seeing the dream and this is something worth being thankful for. The more faculties engaged with the procedure, the better.

At the point when it is difficult to see the desire in one's inner being, it can assist with consolidating it with smelling and feeling things, to see the delight on the essences of others, to hear them state how cheerful they are. To make perceptions – a solid method to change reality rapidly – work, it's implied that you don't need to see the truth in one's imagination, yet the changed and wished reality and to envision oneself in that reality, as though it were valid. As consistent with life and as delineated as could reasonably be expected.

Concentrate this in a picture with the basics, an image of the outcomes acquired. At that point, you can generally bring out that image during the daytime. What one can picture, can turn out to be valid, as it appears that nobody can picture something that can't exist.

I have seen that many affirmations apply to us in daily life and you need to look at these considerations when you are planning to apply affirmations for your weight loss program.

- having confidence in the strategy is required

– it even makes your desire work out quicker than the negligible utilization of affirmations; the blend of the two things is great

- when your confidence has not yet been fortified by confirmations of the strategy or are you still somewhat suspicious, at that point you need to focus on objectives that are simpler to accomplish

- the way that what you wish ought not to hurt anybody or upset another person's desire

- make an exact picture in one's eye's brain, a picture that can be recovered without any problem

- 'see' this picture particularly toward the beginning of the day and at night and attempt to recover it during daytime however many occasions as could be expected under the circumstances, when you are loose

- don't attempt to disentangle how a desire turns out to be valid

- don't burn through your time on the inquiry to what extent it will take, as this diminishes the intensity of the desire.

Understanding Self-Hypnosis and Weight Loss On A Deeper Level

When you understand self-hypnosis and start to implement it in your daily life, you will start to see changes in your body and mind. In this section, I will explain some truths behind this process that will help you clear any doubts that you have regrinding this process. I will not focus on the self-hypnosis in detail as I have covered this topic in the previous chapter will only focus on the relation between weight loss and self-hypnosis.

- Self-hypnosis is a viable method to get to your brain-body association and to convey thoughts and pictures of your ideal body to your inner mind.

There is a plenitude of clinical writing backing the adequacy of hypnosis in affecting physical or brain-body capacities. The examinations accomplished for different ailments exhibit the force and clinical viability of self-hypnosis. You don't need to trust that a hundred additional investigations will be distributed about weight reduction and hypnosis. You can pioneer your path at this moment. Your self-hypnosis can assist you with beating hindrances and reasons by allowing you to pick, and subliminally engage, the thoughts, emotions, convictions, and practices that will deliver the outcomes you need. It can likewise assist you with conquering hindrances and reasons by subliminally following up on your decisions, thoughts, emotions, convictions, and practices that will create the outcomes you need.

- Self-hypnosis lets you utilize the intensity of conviction and acceptance.

By centering and coordinating this force inside the brain-body, your inner mind acknowledges and follows up on your convictions as evident—in any event, when they are deceptions. It has been demonstrated that people can hold confidence at the top of the priority list that lets them stroll over hot coals without making a consume reaction. A virus object that is accepted to be blisteringly hot can be contacted and produce a consume reaction. You can pick what to accept and stimulate it with your confidence or conviction of realizing that it generally will be valid for you. Your self-hypnosis lets you exploit the insight that "It is done unto you as indicated by your confidence." Your brain-body even acknowledges deceptions, since it doesn't recognize what is genuine and what you envision or claim to be genuine. Become aware of what you permit yourself to accept consistently.

- Self-hypnosis lets you reframe and reinvent subliminal examples and reactions so they become predictable with your inspiration, convictions, and assumptions regarding your ideal weight.

A large number of your standards of conduct, food inclinations, and convictions about your weight and yourself were made from the get-go in life before you had the mindfulness and scholarly advancement to settle on decisions about what was being realized in your mind-body. A genuine case of this is the impact that being a perfect plate club part has had on confounding the impressions of yearning, totality, and when to quit eating. Reinventing this example with the conviction that you don't need to clean your plate can enable you to explain when to quit eating. Self-hypnosis lets you fix the mind discovering that followed enthusiastic and awful encounters. Whatever is found out can be unlearned by picking up something different in its place. Your self-hypnosis gives the way to learn propensities and examples that give you the ideal weight results you need. This incorporates eating and yearning designs, food inclinations, the enthusiastic relationship to nourishments and eating, self-picture, the impact of injury, and different subliminal elements influencing you.

- Self-hypnosis gives a variety of instruments (trancelike marvels) that can assist you with accomplishing your ideal weight.

These include: recollecting and overlooking, adjusting tangible observation, time contortion, posthypnotic proposal, and that's only the tip of the iceberg. For instance, you may utilize your self-hypnosis to allot a brilliant taste to nourishments that assist you with accomplishing your ideal weight, and allocate an unwanted taste to food sources that neutralize your ideal weight. Posthypnotic recommendations are one more of the numerous instruments or entrancing marvels accessible to you. You can entrancingly recommend that you will encounter an awesome sentiment of completion part of the way through a supper and leave the rest of. Or on the other hand you may twist time or disregard longings or wants for subverting snacks.

- Self-hypnosis can modify the manner in which you see impediments to making changes in physical action, work out, and different practices that are vital and charming in accomplishing your ideal weight.

It doesn't make a difference if your past has excluded standard examples of physical movement and exercise. That is in the past at this point. Your self-hypnosis can assist you with viewing exercise as attractive and fulfilling. It can help expel the impediments to more prominent physical action by helping you make the demeanor that coordinates the practices to create the outcomes you want.

- Self-hypnosis is a successful method to encounter the antitoxin to push — unwinding.

Self-hypnosis diminishes the pressure related with evolving propensities, perspectives, and practices and can make a compelling boundary and protection to the manners by which stress can influence responsive eating conduct and physical capacity. You can't be loose and restless or worried simultaneously. They are two distinctive physiological states. As you practice your selfhypnosis, your brain body is retaining the capacity to deliver an unwinding reaction. You can trigger the unwinding reaction when you wind up in distressing circumstances that risk your ideal weight. This can go from worry during occasion suppers when others need you to eat gigantic amounts of the food they serve you, to routine work focuses on that you recently quieted by eating something. You can likewise deliver an unwinding reaction when you are amidst evacuating an old propensity and making another one.

- Self-hypnosis can change and divert the solid energies of desires and enticements into sentiments and practices that protect your ideal weight.

Your training with self-hypnosis shows you how to specifically separate or separate from your condition and your inward state. This lets you recall the separated state or become a disconnected spectator and notice that "longings are available"— and afterward pick what to transform that vitality into for your motivations. You don't have to attempt to deny longings and enticement; rather, just disengage from the emotions they deliver and see that they are available. Your self-hypnosis is a brilliant method to practice your capacity to confine all around ok to then pick what you need to understanding. This is likewise one of the manners in which that hypnosis is utilized to make entrancingly initiated sedation.

- Self-hypnosis can assist you with making a progressively pleasurable and adoring relationship with food, eating, and your body, making your weight reduction and way of life changes increasingly successful and charming.

As you make and appreciate more prominent joy with new propensities for eating and physical exercise, you will look after them. A caring relationship with anything lets you make the most of your involvement in it. Your self-hypnosis causes you accomplish the internal work of cherishing that makes the outcomes you need for your ideal weight.

- Self-hypnosis is a type of centered focus that adequately upgrades your capacity to intellectually practice accomplishing the outcomes you want.

Mental practice has been utilized by competitors and entertainers for quite a long time. Studies have demonstrated mental practice to be a powerful method to rehearse one's mind body for the real execution. Your self-hypnosis lets you practice the delight of your exhibition at unique events, occasion meals, and gatherings. You can sleepily practice your food and refreshment decisions, your trust in declining dishes or beverages, and fulfillment in dealing with the circumstance so well indeed. Practicing at the top of the priority list, you are setting up your brain body to serve your ideal weight and joy ahead of time.

- Self-hypnosis successfully empowers the reiteration and practice of sleep inducing recommendations that bring about deep rooted, perpetual examples of conduct, feeling, and conviction about your ideal weight. Whatever you consistently practice with your self-hypnosis will turn into the cognizant and subliminal examples of the way of life that keeps up your ideal weight.

Before you know it, you will hear yourself telling others that you don't need to consider eating less junk food or weight reduction any longer. Your way of life is presently in real life, building up the examples and propensities that produce the outcomes you need. Your self-hypnosis made ready for some progressions while letting you focus on finding and making your own special formula for immaculate weight.

- The Self-Hypnosis Diet isn't an eating regimen.

It gives the missing ingredient that encourages you utilize your brain body to build up deep rooted examples of eating and exercise that cause it to appear as though you can eat anything you need and still keep your ideal weight

Conclusion

After completing this book, you should start reviewing the chapters and start adopting the changes to ensure that you lose weight and have a positive mindset when it comes to your soul and body. People tend to lose sight of the greater good and never follow through with the diet programs. The main problem with most of people is a focus and how they see themselves. The mind is a very powerful tool and you can unlock the potential of the body when you have a clear mind.

All you need to do is to meditate and have positive affirmations when it comes to your body and mind. These will help you get a positive mindset and also adopt the routines that will help you shed the extra pounds easily.

Appendix A

1- Hypnosis is a very complicated process and if you want to learn it, you have to spend many sessions and follow many instructions. This statement is FALSE. Hypnosis is a simple and easy process.

2- You will have to be hypnotized by a person who knows this trade. FALSE. The process of hypnosis can be done by anyone.

3- The person loses touch with his consciousness when he/she is in a hypnotic trance. FALSE. You will not lose consciousness when you are hypnotized.

4- The subconscious mind will not know the difference between the imaginary and real worlds. TRUE. The subconscious mind is a tricky part and you may not differentiate between the real and imaginary things.

5- The hypnosis will let you do unwanted things and you may also violate your values in this process. FALSE. Even when you are hypnotized, you will not lose your values.

6- People go the stage of trance every day. TRUE. Many people experience trance daily.

7- Hypnosis is also known as self-hypnosis. TRUE.

8- The process of hypnosis can help you heal your body. TRUE. Many studies tell us that hypnosis can be used to heal the body.

9- The body has a language and it cannot be understood. TRUE. The body has its very own language but this statement is not entirely true. With some practice, you will be able to understand the signals given by your body.

10-   The process of hypnosis can be used to change the physical responses such as breathing and digestion. TRUE.

11-Medical hypnosis is similar to stage hypnosis. FALSE. While stage hypnosis is used for entertainment, medical hypnosis can be used to heal the body.

12-   Sometimes you will not know when you are in trance. TRUE.

13-   Hypnosis is a mental stage and it just a mental phenomenon. FALSE. The brain scans show that hypnosis has effects on the body as well.

14-   Some people in the world cannot be hypnotized. TRUE.

15-   Hypnosis can be used to give messages from the body to the mind and vice versa. TRUE.

16-   You can easily find thousands of research studies on this topic that can help you evaluate the benefits of hypnosis. TRUE

References

❖ Guiliano, Mireille. French Women Don't Get Fat: The Secret of Eating for Pleasure. New York: Vintage, 2007

❖ O'Driscoll, Erin. The Complete Book of Isometrics: The Anywhere, Anytime Fitness Book. New York: Hatherleigh Press, 2005.

❖ Temes, Roberta. The Complete Idiot's Guide to Hypnosis. 2nd ed. New York: Alpha Books, 2004.

❖ Yano, Jessica M., Kristie Yu, Gregory P. Donaldson, Gauri G. Shastri, Phoebe Ann, Liang Ma, Cathryn R. Nagler, Rustem F. Ismagilov, Sarkis K. Mazmanian, and Elaine Y. Hsiao. "Indigenous Bacteria from the Gut Microbiota Regulate Host Serotonin Biosynthesis." Cell 161 (2015)

❖ Ursell, Luke K., Henry J. Haiser, Will Van Treuren, Neha Garg, Lavanya Reddivari, Jairam Vanamala, Pieter C. Dorrestein, Peter J. Turnbaugh, and Rob Knight. "The Intestinal Metabolome: An Intersection Between Microbiota and Host." Gastroenterology 146 (2014)

❖ Weil, Andrew. Eating Well for Optimum Health: The Essential Guide to Food, Diet, and Nutrition. New York: Knopf, 2000.

CPSIA information can be obtained
at www.ICGtesting.com
Printed in the USA
BVHW051350270421
605941BV00002B/201

9 781802 340556